LIVE
NOURISHED

LIVE NOURISHED

MAKE PEACE *with* FOOD,
BANISH BODY SHAME,
and RECLAIM JOY

SHANA MINEI SPENCE,
MS, RDN, CDN

SIMON ELEMENT

New York   London   Toronto   Sydney   New Delhi

To my parents,
who are the most inspirational humans I know.

CONTENTS

LIVE
NOURISHED

INTRODUCTION

Diet culture [noun]: a system that profits off of unrealistic Eurocentric, thin, and unhealthy ideals and expectations; an industry worth over $70 billion; an ideology that calls itself a lifestyle, a change, a cleanse, a detox in order to disguise that it is really a scam; a philosophy that takes a negative mental toll on its users and leaves chaos in its wake.

Diet culture is a term that is used so frequently throughout media that I think it's important to define what it truly is right at the beginning. After all, *culture* can be interpreted in a number of ways: it can be the customary beliefs, social norms, and material traits of a racial, religious, or social group or the set of shared attitudes, values, goals, and practices that characterizes an institution or organization.[1] With the shared belief (by many in society) that we need to shrink ourselves in order to become better humans both physically and morally, it's pretty apparent that dieting is indeed a culture in itself. Normalizing this even further, diet culture is now frequently referred to as a lifestyle, lending it a positive connotation. But here's the thing about diet culture: It is the opposite of health. Dieting and restriction have so many negative outcomes that there is nothing healthy about them at all.

It is very easy to fall victim to diet culture because it is everywhere, and we are all susceptible. I took a sharp detour from dieting, shrinking, and thinking I was morally superior for being disciplined enough to "take care of myself." In other words, I was in diet hell. In fact, many of us who now talk and write about diet culture have escaped this hell ourselves, and our goal is to help others do the same.

Before we really dive in, I am a Registered Dietitian Nutritionist (RDN), and I also earned a BS degree (yes, bachelor of science, but also the other BS phrase that you're definitely thinking of) in fashion merchandising. I have spent many years in school learning about the science and intricacies of food and the human body, but that doesn't mean that part of those learnings weren't completely biased and stigmatized. But if we rewind to an even earlier part of my life before nutrition, it's easy to see where my introduction to diet culture began.

When I share that I used to work in fashion, I'm usually met by a lot of oohs and aahs. It sounds glamorous and mysterious. Fancy clothes, runway shows, parties, and beautiful people having a great time. And it was exciting, in a way, if your definition of exciting is regularly crying in fashion closets away from the security cameras because the toxicity of the environment was just too much to handle. Glamorous indeed.

During this period of my life, I was so unhappy and miserable because of my job that I didn't realize that same job was triggering disordered eating habits. (I hesitate to label it as an eating disorder because I never received an actual diagnosis, but all the criteria were there.) I was constantly looking in the mirror and thinking I could be thinner, constantly judging my eating habits, plus feeling out of control with my career. Finding ways to control my body was a way for me to cope.

Ever a millennial, I looked to technology for answers and downloaded an app. One in particular taught me a way to restrict my calories to 1,400 a day. It was the perfect bandage for my pain at the time. Was I constantly getting shut down by a manager with daily microaggressions? Yes. But I was also quickly losing weight and feeling superior because I was able to contort my body. Microaggressions can easily be ignored when you're dropping two jean sizes in a month.

Like many people I was young and impressionable, and so I fell for the lies that diet culture was selling. I began meticulously writing down every single morsel of food I put in my mouth, and at the end of the day I would judge myself on how well I did. (Yeah, I know.) I carried a little notebook with me everywhere I went so I could record everything. I weighed myself every morning and recorded that as well. I was so proud of myself as the pounds came off; I really thought I was accomplishing something great—that I was bettering my health. I prided myself on my willpower and ability to resist temptation and hung inspirational photos of celebrities and models around my dorm room. I used all the articles and pictures that I tore from the magazines I collected to fuel my determination to make myself as small as I could. I thought I was being so healthy, and because these tactics were highlighted in the media I was consuming, I also thought this was normal.

During my tenure in fashion, my disordered eating ballooned, coupling severe restriction with orthorexia (an unhealthy focus on healthy eating). I felt the constant need to prove to myself that I was at my most superior level of health. But in actuality, I was miserable and lost, and my body was something I could manipulate and control. Or so I thought. During this time, I also started taking ballet classes. I had taken dance classes since I was a child, and although it never transitioned into something serious, I enjoyed the feeling of movement. I found a studio that was close to my apartment that offered classes in the evenings. There I could feel liberated, even if it was just for a couple of hours. And this feeling of liberation occurred because I was enjoying dance, but I also loved the sense of community that I was gaining. I made friends with other adult women my age whom I started seeing regularly at class. And with extra practice, I was getting really good. Not Misty Copeland–level of professional dance but to the point where I was singled out in class and readily admired. My sun sign is Leo, so while a little self-adoration is of course welcome, there is a reason I'm sharing this.

What goes up must come down. My teacher was this amazing woman whom I admired. A former ballerina from Romania, she treated the class like we were professional dancers. This meant really caring for and paying attention to her students, which was motivating. This was all great for me because I felt as though I was excelling at this beautiful art form that I loved. I was dancing every day and eventually found myself doing triple pirouettes, memorizing choreography, and dancing on pointe, which not only solidified my progress but also contributed to my disordered eating.

Many people associate ballerinas with eating disorders because of the svelte physique the profession is often known for. I soon became very familiar with this feeling myself. "Your legs are lengthening." *Lengthening* is a code word for slimming. It was after class and I was heading out when my teacher casually mentioned this. It was meant as a nonchalant compliment, but for me, this meant my hard work was being noticed and admired. I took it as a challenge. It did not matter at all that I was not an actual ballerina. I was still willing to put my body through a physical toll to attain a certain aesthetic. So as the weight continued to shed through my starvation methods, the compliments I received grew. How could I possibly stop now? It didn't matter that I was obsessing over every morsel of food. It didn't matter that I was sacrificing social aspects of my life (turning down invitations to gatherings and parties) in favor of exercising and due to fear over what food would be served. It didn't matter that I stopped menstruating or that I was getting injured frequently. None of this mattered at the time because I was looking at this lifestyle as a matter of willpower, a sacrifice that I was willing to make. My physical and mental health were slowly declining, but it was all good because I was "slimming and lengthening." This is diet culture 101, a mindset that sees you breaking down physically and mentally but still tells you that the after photo, the transformation, is all that counts. And let's be honest, the after isn't truly an after. It's a during, because diets and restrictions fail at a ridiculously high rate.

Luckily, my story has a happy ending, as eventually I got fed up with this toxic give-and-take. I began realizing this was not what I wanted emotionally, physically, or professionally. The whole experience made me question my life's purpose, and so I started to investigate other career paths, which is how I stumbled onto the field of nutrition science. I started looking up nutrition facts and became interested in what all the hot celebrities were eating and how they were dieting. (And yes, this is the opposite stance that I have on nutrition now, but we all have a learning curve.) I was a Google warrior. At some point, a light bulb turned on, and I realized that I could use my Google skills to become a nutritionist. I liked to eat healthy (what was really orthorexia) and I thought I could, of course, get other people to do the same. Unfortunately, my reasoning for getting into nutrition was not uncommon. Many nutrition professionals get into the field because of an eating disorder or as a way to project their unhealthy habits onto others—in the name of health, of course. This isn't meant to be directly harmful, but it does highlight how influential diet culture is; and in fact, up to 89 percent of nutrition dietetic students meet the criteria for orthorexia.[2] I didn't even know what a dietitian was at the time (please don't laugh), but felt compelled to dictate to others how to eat. I thought that I was going to just get a certificate online and then be able to instruct others.

My parents were the first people I talked to about my career move, and they were *thrilled*. They had hated the fact that I worked in fashion, so their daughter now investigating a career change was a most welcome idea. God bless my mom, who started doing her own research on nutrition careers—like I said, they were ecstatic—and found out there were people called dietitians out there, and that they had legitimate degrees. So, to make this work, not only would I have to go back to school but I would also have to take additional prerequisite classes to get a degree in nutrition. Some further digging revealed that once I graduated, the road only got steeper. According to Google, I would have to try to get into an internship program with a match rate of 49 percent to get experience. And that internship would almost certainly be unpaid. And would probably last close to a year. Then I would have to pass a national exam to be licensed. Well, that six-week nutrition certificate was looking really freaking tempting, let me tell you. But I took the plunge and went all in, in hopes of becoming a dietitian.

While taking my initial courses and learning the basics of how science and nutrition are intertwined, I also started learning about different communities and the differences in how socioeconomic factors can affect health. For instance, I grew up in East Flatbush, Brooklyn, pre-gentrification. Growing up in this neighborhood, I could clearly see the differences in food access and income based on neighborhood lines. East Flatbush is a residential neighborhood and one that is predominantly Black (African American and Caribbean), so much so that in 2017, the neighborhood was officially dubbed the Little Caribbean. With these demographics, there are, unsurprisingly, adverse health outcomes and poverty. Living in neighborhoods with higher rates of poverty limits options and makes it difficult to access quality health care and resources that are health promoting. East Flatbush's unemployment rate is 9 percent, with a 19 percent poverty rate, as of this writing. Access to affordable housing and employment opportunities with fair wages and benefits are also closely associated with good health. More statistics show that 54 percent of East Flatbush residents are rent burdened, which means they pay more than 30 percent of their income for housing and may have difficulty affording food, clothing, transportation, and health care. For every one supermarket, there are twenty-one bodegas in the neighborhood. (For those who are unfamiliar, the bodega can be described as the heart and soul of New York. You want a coffee and a buttered roll on the way to the subway? Stop at the bodega. Do you need to grab a can of corn for a recipe but you're short on time? Stop at the bodega. I have memories of being in middle school and having a dollar and coming out with a flavored water that cost twenty-five cents and a bag of potato chips and a candy bar. Now, that was back in the day in the '90s, so I am dating myself. But I digress.) As great as they are, bodegas do not have the same options and assortment that many supermarkets provide. This is vital, because social determinants of health play a role in health outcomes. Currently, 15 percent of East Flatbush adults have been diagnosed with diabetes, and 36 percent of the adults have hypertension. Stress and trauma from environmental factors play a role in conditions such as diabetes and hypertension.[3]

These numbers can also do the talking when it comes to the disparity of access to equitable care and needs. I've seen it with my own eyes. My mother used to travel once a week to the nearby neighborhood of Park Slope (a twenty-minute drive) just for the more diverse grocery options. Why were things "better" there? Demographically speaking, Park Slope has a higher number of white residents. For every one supermarket, there are twelve bodegas compared to the twenty-one of East Flatbush. And for what it's worth, there aren't just fewer bodegas; there are more supermarkets. Need more stats? Ten percent of Park Slope residents live in poverty and 6 percent are unemployed. Meanwhile, 37 percent are rent burdened compared to the 54 percent in East Flatbush. Looking at health statistics, 6 percent of residents have diabetes and 22 percent have hypertension.[4] And this isn't simply a Brooklyn thing. There are comparisons to be made across the country between primarily white neighborhoods and neighborhoods that mainly house persons of color. I guarantee you that there are hundreds of thousands of similar cases. These are systemic inequities and inequalities that, quite frankly, can be discussed at length in another book, but know that they exist.

So when I went back to school for nutrition and started studying community health, I wasn't surprised to learn about the chronic disease disparities within neighborhoods with very different incomes. I was a firsthand witness to it. While I was writing a paper about this very topic for class, I realized this disparity was at the heart of why I wanted to become a dietitian. I really wanted to make a difference. I had lofty dreams of giving back to my community, intervening in the area of nutrition education, and spurring a movement toward healthier eating. Unfortunately, this meant thinking I would promote weight loss. I believed that weight loss meant making my community healthier because thinner was better. I had BMI (body mass index) ranges and cutoffs memorized down to a tenth of a pound, and I was proud of that. That's the thing with a diet culture mindset: even though you see how certain aspects are unattainable or unsustainable, the narrative of an ideal body is still perpetuated. Thinner = healthier, no matter what. And while I still wanted to help my community, this mindset was steeped in healthism and orthorexia, placing responsibility on the individual. (Healthism is a dangerous belief that situates the problem of health and disease at the level of the individual. Solutions are formulated at that level as well.[5]) Health at Every Size? I'd never heard of it, and even if I had, at the time, I wouldn't have believed it.

Once I started my master's program, I began sinking deeper into diet culture, a way of thinking that was only bolstered by the institution. As with most health professionals, school taught me all about how to stigmatize. Yes, you read that correctly. As part of our coursework, I learned that certain populations are more likely to have certain illnesses and diseases. And my classmates and I typed all these notes into our laptops without a second thought. Of course, we didn't learn that these populations were dealing with little access to health care, systemic racism, low income, weight stigmatization, misogyny, and dozens of other factors that contributed to these illnesses. We left shaking our heads thinking noncompliance, believing that those populations inherently didn't care about their health. Yes, even I, a Black woman, along with other BIPOC folks, believed that we needed to intervene within our cultures because they were the problem. It seems bizarre to me now that I ever thought that way, but when you are an eager student lapping up information from established academic experts, you tend to believe it.

And it's completely understandable to not question these ideas. I'd heard these notions way before I entered a graduate school classroom. We hear messages like this in the media beginning at a young age and we internalize them. And when you hear something repeatedly, you believe it. Think back to watching television shows and seeing which characters were there for the audience to laugh *at*. Television shows and movies love to present the funny fat sidekick character as comedic relief. Think young Monica on *Friends*. Or Fat Amy in *Pitch Perfect*. And the movie series *Big Momma's House*. The constant jokes about their bodies and their eating habits only reinforce what we are told about people in larger bodies, that they are food obsessed and are not to be taken seriously.

Fast forward to me officially receiving a master's degree in ~~diet culture~~ nutrition in 2017 and earning a license in 2018. I was so excited and ambitious and even secured my dream job in public health a few months later. I was on a freaking roll; nothing could stop me. After a year or so, I started posting about nutrition on social media, sort of making it up as I went along. I posted a bunch of what-I-eat-in-a-day pictures. *Cringe*. I posted about all the ways to lose weight. *Harder cringe*. I also posted a bunch of inspirational Pinterest quotes about how we all just need willpower and how it only takes small changes to add up. I'm not making this shit up. However, if proof is needed, all you have to do is scroll through older social media posts from when I was a newbie dietitian. I distinctly remember not really knowing what direction I wanted to take for my career, so I dabbled in everything.

I also started to follow other dietitians to see what they were discussing and posting. Most of their social media posts were like mine, but I noticed a few posts about so-called diet culture. I wanted to know more. I had recovered from my disordered eating (or so I thought). I wasn't counting calories or using an app, but I still was conscious of my intake and thought that dietitians had to have a certain look. But I was sure I was *definitely* over my dieting phase—at least that's what I told myself. We associate dieting with fad diets and calorie counting, but it takes awhile to realize that diet culture has a larger grasp on us than we realize. And back when I was first starting out, I had never thought of dieting as a culture. Sure, I disliked the idea of fad diets like keto or Paleo, but fully letting go of diets altogether wasn't something that was on my radar. I still thought the pursuit of thinness was the same as the pursuit of health and didn't see food restriction as something entirely harmful. So hearing about something called diet culture definitely sparked my curiosity.

In 2019, one of my colleagues casually asked me if I had read *Anti-Diet* by Christy Harrison. *Anti-Diet?* What was that? According to my coworker, it was mind-blowing. I immediately went out and bought Harrison's book. And, well, it was life-changing; it was the first time I had read anything regarding the diet industry and its predatory ways. In short, *Anti-Diet* explains the way our society is programmed to look at health and bodies in a certain way that only benefits the industry. We revere thinness simply because we are told we should. We also don't care how an individual attains this thinness. Just look at the diets that line the pockets of the creators and influencers for proof. Not to mention the medical professionals who recommend invasive surgeries, such as bariatric surgery, without really giving the individual sufficient warnings about the aftermath. I don't think I put the book down once I started reading. I slowly began to understand what diet culture encompassed and how engrossed in it we were as a society. This culture was very much an industry, and what keeps industries thriving is money. I realized the money I spent on apps, books, and memberships was all a part of the vicious cycle of dieting. The subtitle of *Anti-Diet* is *Reclaim Your Time, Money, Well-Being, and Happiness Through Intuitive Eating*. The more I thought of this, the closer to home it felt.

Diet culture is a life thief, posits Harrison, as it steals the joy and spark of everyday living. And she's so right. I thought about how miserable I was during my restricting years. I felt like a zombie just going through the motions of looking up the calories of every food and plugging them into my app like clockwork. Even if I had only eaten half a grape, you better believe I was documenting that half grape. Then making sure I was including all my movement. My ballet classes were fun, yes, but they were also a means to earn all my food and make up for everything I ate. Reading *Anti-Diet* made me really reflect on all the years of dieting. It made me reflect on not only the money but also the time that I spent calculating and weighing my food. The time I lost with loved ones because I was so consumed with my disordered habits on this quest to be the absolute thinnest I could be, all because society told me that was ideal. This was also the first time I realized that the BMI system is flawed and heard the phrase Health at Every Size (HAES). That's when it hit me: Although I was a licensed dietitian, I had received a degree in diet culture. I knew I had to change my perspective and my approach to helping people.

During my initial job hunt after I received my license, my goal was to begin working in public health. (As of this writing, I work for a New York City government agency providing nutrition education.) In the very beginning of my time, I was teaching with a thinner-is-better mindset, with a healthism and elitist attitude. After reading *Anti-Diet*, doing my own thorough research on the topic of HAES, and immersing myself in the context and language of the movement, I realized it was time for me to change how I thought, spoke, and taught. I will also say that I am still constantly learning and evolving, because no one is perfect. There is always more to be said and learned.

Harrison's book was the stepping stone for how I now approach counseling and my ideology surrounding a healthy relationship with food, but there are still some elements missing when discussing diet culture. With my experience working in public health, as well as my lived experience from growing up in East Flatbush as a Black woman, I can add layers and intersectionality to the idea of diet culture. It took awhile for me to grasp the simple concept that as health professionals, we shouldn't assess health based on looks and size; much of health is out of our control, and so much of what is discussed in the media is based on healthism. When you get a degree in diet culture, it's hard to comprehend how to not assess health based on numbers and body size.

From a young age, we watch television, we read magazines, we see advertisements. We are immersed in a society telling us what we should look like and aspire to be. You don't have to be a health professional to have preconceived ideas that thinner is better and that people are in charge of their own health. This is all part of the media that we consume and the ideas that we constantly see. If you see something enough times, you don't question it. It's part of the programming we are fed since childhood. But in my work with private clients, I have found that it makes an enormous difference to approach a nutrition session with behavior modifications and changes such as adding nutrient-dense foods, finding ways to reduce stress, and increasing bouts of joyful movement instead of just reacting to numbers on a scale. When I first started counseling using this approach, I would ask myself, *How would I counsel if this was a thin person?* I would never base any behavior modifications on body size. And contrary to popular belief, not focusing on numbers is actually health promoting because it doesn't have the same physical and mental toll that straight-up restriction does. Not to mention, a large portion of really getting to the root of the issue is asking someone about their current lifestyle and not assuming anything. Too often health professionals will prejudge based on learned stereotypes instead of the actual issue in front of them. Don't assume that someone isn't exercising. Don't assume that someone isn't eating whole grains or vegetables. Don't assume someone has a chronic illness or condition based on their physical appearance. Health neither has a specific look nor dictates someone's morality.

Using these tactics and methods, I have noticed a change in clients' responses and levels of comfort. Their stress levels are noticeably decreased and their level of trust increases. I am a health professional who looks at my clients as people, not numbers, and listens to them as such. In our first session, one client remarked, amazed, on how I hadn't asked for their weight. Instead of watching the numbers on the scale, I work with clients to establish a healthy relationship with food, because the disordered habits that we as a society normalize (food restriction, overexercising, skipping meals, using supplements as hunger replacements, and more) are so engrained in us. It shouldn't be mind-blowing to counsel someone that it's okay to eat and nourish themselves, but because restriction is normalized, it can feel profound.

I do want to point out that I took the time to learn these things because I was open-minded. I don't blame health professionals or even non–health professionals who aren't fully onboard with weight inclusivity. We've all been taught about diet culture from a young age, whether we realize it or not. But while it's an understandable mindset, that doesn't mean this way of thinking can't or shouldn't change. As a rebuttal to weight inclusivity, I constantly hear, "But a dietitian should care about health." And I always answer, "Yes, exactly!" Because my approach in both my practice and in this book *is* focused on health, in a way that is so much less stressful and, ultimately, so much more freeing.

What I hope you get out of *Live Nourished* is a better understanding of a weight-inclusive approach to living and how to dismantle diet culture not only for yourself but also for others you can educate. You're going to learn about the racist, capitalist, and patriarchal history (and current reality) of diet culture so you can see it for what it is. You're going to realize that we don't have to earn anything, because we need food to survive. You're going to learn exactly *why* diets never work (hint: it's got nothing to do with willpower, and more to do with the body's reaction to moving in and out of starvation mode, as well as its reaction to stress, including trauma). You're going to learn how to create a positive and joyful relationship with food that is both healthy and sustainable. If we can each individually shift our thinking, together as a society we can break away from the toxicity of diet culture and live freely and healthily in our bodies.

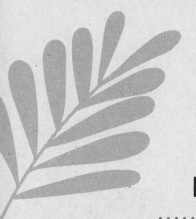

PART ONE

· ·

THE DIET CULTURE TRAP

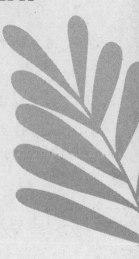

CHAPTER ONE

WHY DIETS DON'T WORK

The stress of dieting does more damage to the body than a cookie ever will.

We hear it thrown around all the time, but have you ever actually thought about what the word *diet* means? Well, it has certainly strayed from its true definition. The origin of the word comes from the Greek *diaita*, which means "a way of living"; more specifically, it signifies a way of living as advised by a physician, which could include food consumption and other daily habits. The word *diet* first appeared in the English language in the thirteenth century and, when used then, referred to the food and drink that we humans ingest.[1] Today, *Merriam-Webster* defines it as 1. food and drink regularly provided or consumed; 2. habitual nourishment; 3. the kind and amount of food prescribed for a person or animal for a special reason; and 4. a regimen of eating and drinking sparingly so as to reduce one's weight.[2] None of these definitions are technically incorrect, but it is sort of mind-blowing that generally today, the final definition—the one that is ranked lowest and that is the most negative—is the one most commonly used.

• THE ENDLESS DIET CYCLE •

Whether we like it or not, diets are now synonymous with re-striction and control. Whether it's restricting a certain item or limiting a particular food group, the common theme of mod-ern diets is taking something away or labeling something as bad. There's a bunch of different ways that this can manifest: Cutting out carbohydrates, or sugar (which, yes, is a carb), or fat. Eating less than an adequate number of calories. Only con-suming food between certain hours of the day. And on and on. If you were to ask someone who is still locked in the clutches of diet culture what their food intake looked like, they will very quickly tell you about keto or Whole30 or intermittent fasting, and list all the foods they aren't allowed to eat and the hours during which they can eat. It's very likely they are well versed in this language because this is probably not the first diet they have tried.

Don't think diets are that common? In 2020, the Centers for Disease Control and Prevention (CDC) reported that in 2015–18, 17.1 percent of US adults aged twenty and over were on a special diet.[3] The rate of dieting women was higher than dieting men, at 19 percent versus 15.1 percent. One thing to note is that the participants of this study were asked if they were on any kind of diet either to lose weight or address another health concern. The special diets were slotted into the following cate-gories: weight loss or low-calorie diets, low-fat or low-cholesterol diets, low-sodium diets, sugar-free or low-sugar diets, low-fiber diets, high-fiber diets, diabetic diets, low-carbohydrate diets, and high-protein diets, among others. No surprise, weight loss or low-calorie diets were the most common. The percentage of adults on a special diet also increased in correlation to those who were a higher weight and a higher educational level and was highest among non-Hispanic whites. Now remember, these statistics were for 2015–18. With the rise in social media and access to information now even more readily available, these numbers are almost sure to have increased since then. Not to mention that these stats come from self-reported data from the participants. I mention this because often we don't realize when we are partaking in restrictive habits because Western society has normalized restriction for the sake of health. Meaning that the percentage might actually be much larger.

But why are so many people on weight-loss diets? Well, because diets do work . . . but they also don't. Let me clarify: if we are talking short-term weight loss or that honeymoon phase when the pounds are seamlessly coming off, then yes, they work. You will lose weight initially, but if we're talking long term, no, diets usually don't work. Why? Because diets are not sustainable. Studies have consistently shown that most people regain the weight they have lost and more through dieting. If we look at the numbers, 80 to 95 percent of dieters gain back the weight that they've lost mostly within a year.[4] That's not a promising percentage. If we were prescribed a medication that had an 80 percent chance of *not* working and had the side effects of stress, a risk of developing eating disorders, increased cardiovascular risks, and increased insulin resistance, we certainly wouldn't take it. So why would we want to take those odds by starting a diet?

I'll never forget an interaction I had with someone on social media. I was posting my usual spiel about how restriction is the exact opposite of healthy, and per usual, someone disagreed and felt the need to prove their righteousness to me. These are the CliffsNotes of said interaction:

Them: You're wrong, diets do work.

Me: Okay, if that's what you believe, but I pointed out reasons that they don't for most people.

Them: I lost weight when I was in Weight Watchers (WW) years ago and now I'm doing Noom, which is helping me control myself.

Me: ???

Now, do I believe that social media is the place for constructive arguments and nuance? No. Do I usually entertain these types of "conversations" where the person is not intent on listening? Also no. But I couldn't help but laugh at this interaction, because without even realizing it, this person was proving my point. They mentioned the word *diets*. Diets as in plural, more than one. If diets worked, there wouldn't be a need for you to try a new one every month or year. Not to mention when you are properly nourishing yourself and have a great relationship with food, posts such as these shouldn't be triggering—you shouldn't have to write "I need help with control." You shouldn't need to argue for diet culture on social media at all. But I digress.

When we purchase a product and realize it's not working, we usually don't use it anymore. Yet with diets, we keep at it, even though it's not working. We ignore the constant cycling and the feelings of stress and anxiety because we keep telling ourselves that eventually we will reap the rewards of thinness and happiness and health. Think of it as the perennial dangling carrot, urging us to run forever after it, always trying to reach it and always failing to grab it. But we keep going after it, trying and failing over and over. And this is a universal Western activity. A poll in the United Kingdom of two thousand people found that the average person will try 126 fad diets over the course of their lifetime, and that they will embark on at least two fad diets a year, which typically last just six days each.[5]

But why do we even put ourselves through this in the first place? One of the most common reasons people embark on a weight-loss journey is to better their "health." (I put health in quotations because in reality, health is subjective and very much tailored to the individual. More on this later.) At least that is what dieters believe they are doing, because it is what they've been told by society or even instructed by a health professional. As someone working in health care myself, I know that professionals are just as susceptible to believing that weight loss equals health. Dietitians get their degrees in diet culture, including the class Fatphobia 101. We go to school and learn that seemingly every disease is correlated to a higher weight and also that everyone has full control over their health. This makes many in the field quickly prescribe weight loss as the answer to all problems. But the key word here is *correlation*. And that's not the same as *causation*.

There is no disease or illness that only presents in larger bodies. So, what are people in thinner bodies prescribed for the same illnesses? It's certainly not weight loss. In a 2013 review, researchers reviewed the health outcomes of long-term studies and whether weight-loss diets led to improved cholesterol, triglycerides, systolic and diastolic blood pressure, and fasting blood glucose.[6] Overall, there were only slight improvements in most of the health outcomes studied. Changes in cholesterol, triglyceride levels, blood pressure, and blood glucose were small, and *none* of those changes correlated with weight change because there were health behavior changes, such as in eating pattern, medication use, and exercise. Yes, really.

• YOUR BODY ON A DIET •

We already know that diets more often than not cause the dieter to gain back weight, but that's not the only downside. Simply put, the human body doesn't know the difference between a diet and starvation. So, when you start cutting calories, the body goes into survival mode. Enter our hunger hormones. The hormone leptin, which normally controls levels of satiety, or fullness, decreases. At the same time, levels of the hunger hormone, ghrelin, increase.[7] Ghrelin is produced in our gut and travels through the bloodstream to the brain, where it signals our brain that "Hey, we're hungry, please feed us." Ghrelin levels typically rise before a meal, when your stomach is empty, and decrease shortly after, when your stomach is full. These hormones' main function therefore is to increase appetite, so when we are restricting our intake, our body thinks we're starving, and in true badass body fashion, tries to help by making us feel hungrier. And no, willpower cannot suppress this physiological response. Our bodies are literally fighting to keep us alive and take care of us. They sense danger and are doing everything in their power to protect us from succumbing to a famine state. Kind of cool when you think about it.

So our bodies are actively working against any sort of diet. The most notorious study of our bodies on diets was the Minnesota Starvation Experiment.[8] This clinical study was performed at the University of Minnesota between November 19, 1944, and December 20, 1945. The experiment's primary goal was to examine the physical and psychological effects of prolonged semistarvation on healthy men, as well as the dietary refeeding rehabilitation from this condition. The men were to lose 25 percent of their normal body weight. Each participant spent the first three months of the study eating a normal diet of 3,200 calories a day, followed by six months of semistarvation at 1,570 to 1,800 calories a day, then a restricted rehabilitation refeeding period of three months eating 2,000 to 3,200 calories a day, and finally an eight-week unrestricted rehabilitation period during which there were no limits on caloric intake. The men were also required to work fifteen hours per week, walk twenty-two miles per week, and participate in educational activities for twenty-five hours a week.[9] (It is notable that this normal 3,200 calorie diet would nowadays be considering overeating, and the semistarvation diet of 1,570 calories would be considered normal.)

As you might expect, there were noticeable changes among the men during the semistarvation phase. On the physical end, in addition to their emaciated appearances, there were significant decreases in their strength and stamina, body temperature, heart rate, and sex drive. Psychologically, hunger made the men obsessed with food. They would dream and fantasize about food, read and talk about food, and savor the two meals a day they were given. During this period, the men also reported fatigue, irritability, depression, and lethargy. Interestingly, the men also reported decreases in cognitive ability, although mental testing proved otherwise. (It's worth mentioning that, during the study, out of the thirty-six total participants, three men were excluded because they broke their diet, and a fourth was excluded for not meeting expected weight-loss goals. Yep, diets are universally unsustainable.) Any of this sound familiar? Because I'm pretty sure that anyone who has ever dieted has experienced these same effects.

Many people say they are getting healthier by losing weight and going on a diet. But you have to wonder, is the constant worrying about what you eat and if it's good for you healthy?

Because it seems to be the *exact opposite* of health. You decide to embark on said diet, which is already putting pressure on yourself. You are given an exhaustive list of dos and don'ts that you have to follow in order to succeed. And it really doesn't matter the exact diet you are following, because if it has a set of rules, it is by definition a diet. This can be extremely stressful, especially when we are made to believe that success is the make-it-or-break-it criterion for our health.

To compound this even more, what effect does stress have on the body? The ongoing stress of dieting can cause a fight-or-flight response in the body, causing epinephrine (adrenaline) and cortisol to be released and making us feel more irritable and anxious. Cortisol is a hormone that, under normal circumstances, is released when we're waking up in the morning, exercising, and during small stressful situations like a hard exam, running late to work due to traffic, etc. These situations are usually temporary. Once the "threat" has passed, our hormone levels should return to normal. Another reason that our bodies are really cool: they assist us without us even realizing it. Our parasympathetic nervous system—which is a really fancy way of saying the "automatic system," as in the system that functions automatically—is a network of nerves that relaxes our body after periods of stress or danger and is responsible for the bodily functions that we don't ever think about, such as heart rate, blood pressure, digestion, urination, and sweating, among other functions. This automatic system turns off and is suppressed when we are in a constant state of stress.

Just as our body has a parasympathetic nervous system, it also has a sympathetic nervous system, which puts our body on high alert. Long-term activation of the stress response system and the overexposure to cortisol can negatively impact almost all the body's processes, causing increased risk of many health problems, including but not limited to anxiety, depression, digestive problems, headaches, insomnia, muscle tension and pain, heart disease, heart attack, high blood pressure, and stroke.[10] Notice that this is a lot of bad leading to worse, which really is not good.

• YO-YO DIETING •

Diet culture has really done a number on us. Despite the health risks, we continue to uphold it. Why? Well, vanity says that a thinner aesthetic is preferable, and we are told to do everything possible to get to that aesthetic. This is the reason so many of us have tried multiple diets throughout our lifetime (hello, Oprah). We lose weight and then gain it back, most of the time gaining more weight than we originally started with. Weight cycling, or yo-yo dieting, is defined as losses and subsequent regains of body weight typically occurring in association with weight-loss dieting. As mentioned before, around 80 percent of people who lose weight will gradually regain it to end up at the same weight or even heavier than they were before they went on a diet.[11] Not to mention, the long-term adverse health consequences of weight cycling can include an increased risk for eating disorders, other psychological disorders, and multiple comorbidities including type 2 diabetes, hypertension, cancer, bone fractures, and increased mortality.[12]

What makes it a cycle? Well, it follows some semblance of the below:

- Step 1: You are made to believe that something is wrong with your body and the only way to fix it is through dieting.

- Step 2: You decide to embark on the diet that you heard about through a friend, colleague, aunt, wellness influencer, etc., because if it worked for them, that must mean it will work for you.

- Step 3: The pounds seamlessly come off and the victorious feeling sets in.

- Step 4: You realize that you are becoming more preoccupied with food, thinking constantly about the foods on the list of restrictions. You are also starting to feel stress and anxiety around maintaining the diet.

- Step 5: You start to allow yourself indulgences or cheat days on said foods.

- Step 6: The feeling of giving up is setting in because the cheat days are becoming more consistent, and you feel as though you are becoming obsessed with food.

- Step 7: You start regaining weight.

- Step 8: You begin convincing yourself that this time will be different because you will have more willpower.

- Step 9: You start a new diet. This one will work for sure.

Now, I want to make something *super* clear: I do not use or encourage the use of the terms *indulge* (unless we're talking about purchasing an expensive pair of shoes), *cheat* (unless we're talking about infidelity or copying someone's exam), or *willpower* (because it's not a superpower), nor do I think anyone's body is in need of fixing. I'm including these steps because they illustrate the reason that diets "work," but they really don't. Diet culture thrives on making us believe that something is wrong with our body, and the only way to fix it is to intentionally contort ourselves. But when our efforts to contort don't work, it is us. We are the problem, not the system itself. This is incredibly wrong and a scam that diet culture plays over and over again.

• THE PIPELINE OF DIETS •
TO EATING DISORDERS

Not every diet creates an eating disorder, but there is a noticeable pipeline from dieting to eating disorders. According to the National Eating Disorders Association (NEDA), eating disorders are serious but treatable mental and physical illnesses that can affect people of all genders, ages, races, religions, ethnicities, sexual orientations, body shapes, and weights.[13] What does this have to do with dieting? When we are dieting, we are using restrictive methods and often disordered eating habits; disordered eating is defined as having irregular behaviors surrounding eating that do not meet the diagnostic criteria for an eating disorder as defined by the *Diagnostic and Statistical Manual of Mental Disorders* (*DSM*). According to the Academy of Nutrition and Dietetics, disordered eating symptoms can include

- Chronic weight fluctuations;

- Frequent dieting, anxiety associated with specific foods or meal skipping;

- Rigid rituals and routines surrounding food and exercise;

- Feelings of guilt and shame associated with eating;

- Preoccupation with food, weight, and body image that negatively impacts quality of life;

- A feeling of loss of control around food, including compulsive eating habits; and

- Using exercise, food restriction, fasting, or purging to "make up for bad foods" consumed.[14]

Notice any similarities between these symptoms of disordered eating and dieting? We call it willpower when we decide to miss social events because the food being served might not be on our list of approved foods. We take the blame when we start craving the foods that we are restricting, calling ourselves "obsessed" and "addicted." We have become so accustomed to disordered habits that we don't even recognize them as disordered. Fearing food to the point of counting every single morsel and feeling stress over possibly going over your allotted amount is not healthy.

We get so wrapped up in the promises of diet culture and the quick-fix mentality that we often ignore the effects and the toll dieting has on us. Think about those advertisements for medications that list all the ways taking this simple pill will cure everything, but then at the end very quickly divulge the never-ending list of risks that may make someone think twice about taking it. This is analogous to when someone starts a diet and also ignores the problems that come with it. How have we normalized writing down every morsel of food that we put in our mouths? How have we normalized implying that one food or food group is the root cause of our problems? How have we normalized skipping social events and feeling isolation from fear of food? And most alarming, how is it that we as a society are so concerned with gaining weight and scared of an "obesity epidemic," but we simply shrug at eating disorders and the increasing number of people who suffer from them? Because we are sold lies from diet culture, and since fatphobia (which diet culture stems from) has also been ingrained in our minds, we don't seem to mind working tirelessly in an attempt to contort our bodies to fit a mold.

• EATING DISORDERS • AND DISORDERED EATING

The tactics that we use to contort our bodies very often qualify as disordered eating. This includes use of diet pills, laxatives, purging, bingeing in conjunction with excessive exercising, and food restriction. A quick note on terms here: disordered eating does not automatically equate to an eating disorder since not all behaviors meet the diagnostic criteria from the *DSM*.[15] Further, there is also orthorexia nervosa, which isn't formally recognized in the *DSM* but describes an obsession with healthy eating.[16] This can mean checking ingredient lists in order to determine the healthiness of a food, cutting out food groups, being unwilling to consume anything that isn't "pure" or "healthy," showing distress when healthy options aren't present, and much more. The similarities between orthorexia and anorexia nervosa include development of food preferences, inherited differences in taste perception, food neophobia or pickiness, and a history of parental eating disorders. Even without the *DSM* diagnosis, disordered eating is still extremely problematic and should be addressed with the help of a qualified medical professional. The symptoms might not be as extreme as those with a diagnosable eating disorder, but it is possible for individuals with disordered eating to develop full-blown eating disorders.

Eating disorders are complex diseases that do not discriminate by race, gender, age, or socioeconomic background. There are many factors that can cause eating disorders, including biological risk factors such as genetics and family history. Those who have a family history of mental illness are more likely to also experience mental illness, and diagnoses such as depression, anxiety, or substance use commonly occur with eating disorders.[17] Unlike what we see portrayed in the media, most people with an eating disorder are not underweight, wealthy, and white. Because of that stereotype, there are many people who are not considered sick enough to receive treatment or don't believe they have a problem. But an individual can experience a severe eating disorder at any weight.

While eating disorders and disordered eating are more common in females, we are becoming more aware of a growing number of males who also seek help for eating disorders. Numerous male celebrities are opening up and telling their stories, helping to bring this serious issue to the limelight. Actor Channing Tatum revealed on *The Kelly Clarkson Show* regarding his *Magic Mike* physique that "It's hard to look like that. Even if you do work out, to be that kind of in shape is not natural." Tatum said, "That's not even healthy. You have to starve yourself. I don't think when you're that lean it's actually healthy."[18] While I'm not diagnosing Tatum or suggesting a disorder, the pressure that Hollywood can exert to obtain a certain physique, no matter how harmful the methods used, is not limited to women only. In the United States alone, eating disorders will affect 10 million males at some point in their lives.[19] But due in large part to cultural bias, they are much less likely to seek treatment for their eating disorders. Men are also more likely to be focused on building muscle rather than on weight loss (purging via exercise and misusing steroids).

Women of color are another underrepresented group when it comes to not only recognizing eating disorders but also seeking treatment. This isn't necessarily due to body-image struggles (though this can very well be the case, because demographics are not monoliths) but because women of color suffer from an increase in stress from discriminatory social structures.[20]

Eating disorders are the sum of many stressors. They may be, in part, a response to environmental stress such as abuse, racism, poverty, and/or other environmental factors. For many cultures, weight and body are normal topics at the dinner table and a way that some family members attempt to show love, either through what they think is lighthearted humor—"Every time I see you, you keep getting bigger!"—or by inquiring about health in relation to someone's size or body: "Do you really think you need to be eating that?" But intent doesn't equal outcome, and these triggering scenarios can lead to eating disorders. What some might perceive as harmless comments or suggestions can be dangerous depending on whose ears they fall on. We often receive mixed messages as well, such as "Finish everything on your plate, but don't eat too much"; "You are so beautiful and would be even prettier if you lost weight"; "If you don't ask for seconds, you're going to insult your grandma. Wait—you're taking *another* helping?" Family dynamics could also mean growing up with food insecurity or a lack of access to food. Social media can play a role, too. We are bombarded with images of what we should strive for and what we should want to look like. When we see something enough times, the message being passed down is "You should want to look like this." The more we see these visuals, the more we internalize these messages.

Psychological factors such as perfectionism, distorted body image, and/or past or present traumas are also leading factors in eating disorders.[21] Perfectionism has many layers, which include the pursuit of high standards and critical self-evaluation. High rates of perfectionism are found in anxiety disorders and depression, and perfectionism is significantly associated with anxiety and depression in those with eating disorders.[22] While feeling the need to micromanage and obsessively track food intake and exercise excessively does not *always* cause eating disorders, it never helps with building a healthy relationship with food. Tracking food intake is essentially calorie counting rebranded as something cool—a move right out of the classic diet culture playbook.

CHAPTER TWO

THE HAMSTER WHEEL OF DIET CULTURE

Check in: What will actually make you feel better? A: shedding pounds however you can, or B: figuring out a way to add more nutrients and to eat consistently and in a specific way to nourish your individual body?

In my practice, I've had to ask a lot of clients the above question. It's not surprising, as we are told that thinness is healthy no matter what, and that we should do everything in our power to get to the virtuous status of health. This means entering the never-ending hamster wheel of dieting.

Before we dissect the wheel, take out a pen and put a check mark next to each of the following diets you have tried.

☐ Cigarette diet   ☐ Grapefruit diet

☐ Hollywood diet   ☐ SlimFast

☐ Weight Watchers   ☐ Jenny Craig

☐ Cookie Diet   ☐ Liquid diet

☐ Scarsdale Diet   ☐ Low-fat foods

☐ Cabbage soup diet   ☐ Zone diet

☐ Blood type diet   ☐ Special K diet

☐ Subway diet   ☐ Paleo

☐ Atkins diet   ☐ Keto

☐ South Beach Diet   ☐ Optavia

How many did you check off? I'm willing to guess that not only did you check off one but you likely checked off multiple options, as the ones listed are just some of the more popular diets through the years (1920s–present). We have already covered the scientific reasons why diets don't usually work; however, there is also a capitalist reason they don't usually work.

Let's start by following the money. In 2021, the weight-loss industry in the United States was reportedly worth over $72.6 billion, a sum that is only expected to grow.[1] That is a ton of money to be made. And its unsustainability is the key to a profit, because there is more money to be made with a repeat customer who will keep coming back and spending money in order to alleviate a "problem." We know how diet culture works:

1. Society creates a problem to fix, one that is rooted in fatphobia and really has nothing to do with health.

2. The diet industry decides to solve the problem with costly weight-loss memberships, apps, pills, and books on how to restrict and overexercise.

3. The options presented to solve this problem are not sustainable for individuals. (This is intentional, because if they were, then the industry would burn itself out and there would be no more money to be made.)

4. Individual goes off diet due to unrealistic expectations.

5. Individual feels guilt and shame, as if they did something wrong.

6. Individual decides to restart (or try a new) diet.

7. Repeat forever.

It's a hamster wheel that's hard to get off.

• DIET CULTURE IS EVERYWHERE •

Anyone can fall victim to the grasp of diet culture because the pursuit of unrealistic ideals is so normalized in society. In our current #hustleculture, dieting and restricting are correlated with discipline and being as small as you can be, with taking up less space and being obedient. It's a sign of hard work, of conforming correctly. Any demographic can be targeted. I remember growing up and hearing my father talk about gaining ounces. Yes, that man swore he could tell when he gained ounces. My father was also an athlete, having run track in high school and multiple marathons as an adult, and practiced and competed in martial arts. Like my dad, many athletes are acutely aware of subtle changes in their bodies, since their bodies are their instruments. This only compounds as many athletes are weighed, especially in sports that require competition within a weight class. There are many sports that ask athletes to be smaller and weigh less and also require their bodies to look a certain way physically. And while it may not seem like it on the outside, this is another example of diet culture. Diet culture is not just society telling you to be thinner because it will look better, it's also a coach or an athletic director telling you to be thinner in order to perform better. This in turn can cause many athletes to partake in disordered eating habits, no matter how dangerous. The message is always clear—take up less space. You'd better be obedient as well.

And since obedience is a dictum of the patriarchy, it's really not surprising that so many of these mainstream diets and programs have been founded by men. The "many" here is really a shoutout to Jean Nidetch, the founder of Weight Watchers and one of the few women to start a major diet brand. Dieting and wanting to be as small as possible is all about control: it has roots in anti-fatness, of course, but also in white patriarchy and anti-Blackness. It's a very distinct pipeline, one we will be going into more detail about in a later chapter.

But first, let's take a moment to delve a bit more into Weight Watchers, rebranded as WW, which reported revenue of $1.04 billion in 2022.[2] Yes, $1.04 BILLION. As a child of the nineties, I remember Weight Watchers well. Not because anyone in my family was taking part, but I remember the commercials, the advertisements, and teachers and other adults repeatedly talking about it. In high school, some of the girls brought in their parents' WW books that discussed and categorized all the points that different foods were worth, and then consequently analyzed their lunch choices. We were teenagers thinking about college applications, prom, and who was the cuter boy band, NSYNC or the Backstreet Boys, but we still found time to compute points and critique our bodies. We spent hours scrutinizing our bodies and finding imperfections that we wanted so desperately to fix. And, of course, I wasn't immune to any of these feelings. Remember, this was the era of Britney Spears and Christina

Aguilera and *America's Next Top Model*, with its panel of judges dissecting every inch of the female contestants' thin bodies. Diet culture was everywhere.

Diet culture does not care about the methods that are used, as we can see from the numerous diets that have been created and popularized through the years. It doesn't care about the harmful aftereffects such as stress, the risk of developing eating disorders, increased cardiovascular risks, and increased insulin resistance (which we covered in chapter 1). It only cares about the end result of shrinking the body. And for many folks, this is not actually the end result but the now, because our bodies go through endless weight cycling and the weight loss is not permanent.

We live in a society that uplifts thinness so much that it isn't a surprise many people go through great lengths to contort themselves. And I just have to give my disclaimer that weight loss isn't inherently bad, and there are some people who do lose weight permanently with a diet. This discussion isn't about those people; it is about using dangerous and ultimately ineffective methods. The fact is, these tactics are not often seen as unnecessary or dangerous—they are seen as being disciplined and having willpower. Diet culture subtly affirms that our physical and mental health are just unfortunate casualties in our quest for our desired body.

Our desired body is the result of the problems that are created by society, and then solutions to these problems are created for a profit. A perfect example of this is cellulite, which we are told is unsightly and abnormal. Cellulite is what occurs when the skin overlying certain areas of fat is pulled downward to deeper tissues by connective tissue bands.[3] This creates an uneven surface. As scary as it sounds, it's extremely common and normal to have. Even with this normalcy, there are numerous gels, creams, treatments, and, yes, diets that claim to fix the "problem." But there is no problem, and we've known that for a while. The *Washington Post* published an article in 1985 titled "The Cellulite Myth" in which Dr. Neil Solomon was quoted as saying "There is no such thing as cellulite. And since there is no cellulite, there is no specific treatment for it . . . nothing magical you can take that's suddenly going to make lower body fat disappear."[4]

So how did this term originate and cause such panic among mostly cis women? In 1873, doctors Émile Littré and Charles-Philippe Robin added the word *cellulite* in the twelfth edition of the *Dictionnaire de Médecine*. *Vogue* first printed the term *cellulite* in April 1968, "engendering both a new word *and* a fashionable new way for American women to hate their bodies."[5] Case in point: society creates a problem—in this case, cellulite. Society implies that we should buy into fixes for this problem. And hence diet culture wins again. A Google search of "how to fix cellulite" will bring up numerous and pricey solutions. It's overwhelming to think about the various ways we are taught to be dissatisfied with our appearance in some capacity. It doesn't happen overnight, but with articles, television shows, movies, books, social media, and any other form of media we are consistently consuming. Because of this dissatisfaction, we look for quick fixes to problems that don't need fixing to begin with.

• PURSUIT OF THE THIN IDEAL •

Despite the prevalence of diet culture in our society, there is pushback against the unrealistic ideals and expectations. The body positivity movement is a great example of realizing that the idea of perfection fed to us by the media is ridiculous. Scrolling on social media, you will see images of people showing that bodies come in different varieties and that it is, in fact, normal. However, and this is a big however, this movement still primarily uplifts white, thin, cishet individuals. Anyone can have body dysmorphia, but it is important to know that body dysmorphia often stems from fatphobia. If we weren't constantly fed the fear and negative view of fat bodies, we wouldn't have this sort of body dysmorphia in the first place.

So much of fatphobia is driven by how folks in larger bodies are treated. That mistreatment starts in health care. So much advice is not only weight loss driven but also stems from medical equipment and devices not being made for larger bodies, giving inaccurate readings and results when measuring folks who aren't the white, thin norm. For example, pulse oximeters give inaccurate readings for darker skin.[6] And that finding was made in recent years; so my point is, maybe it's time to realize that many of our health standards should be revised (I will be discussing BMI in the next chapter) because many are driven by Eurocentric standards.

My stance personally is to give advice based on the individual and warnings on certain actions. I will never tell someone that it is wrong to want to lose weight, because I understand where the desire comes from. I always say that I am a non-diet dietitian. I'm not anti-dieter. I will not chastise someone who is primarily interested in losing weight, but I will never recommend fad diets or unnecessary restrictions, either. I treat weight loss like medication and advise on the unpleasant and dangerous side effects of it. I disclose the mental and physical toll it has on the body and will dig deeper to find out what motivations are behind the desire for weight loss. Is it really for health? For example, if someone comes to me with type 2 diabetes, losing weight will not automatically equate to a lower A1C test result because

1. Thin folks can also get type 2 diabetes.

2. Losing weight is not addressing the actual behaviors that someone can take in order to help lower their blood sugar numbers.

This is why I always suggest health-adjusting behaviors— more on those in a bit—that can actually help improve our outcomes and values without sacrificing our relationship to food.

• GO BIG OR GO HOME? •

Thanks to diet culture, we often make the mistake of wanting to do a complete 180 and change everything about our health. Let me be clear that there's nothing wrong with wanting or trying to obtain certain goals, but let's also be clear about the difference between a desire for thinness and a desire for health. Health isn't and shouldn't be a dirty word. But often health is not completely in our control. For some people, ideal health isn't attainable because of a combination of genetic, systemic, and environmental barriers.

While we might not be able to attain society's standard of health, we can, however, attempt to work toward a health goal that is within our individual reach. It's certainly not by throwing out all the foods with added sugar from the fridge. It's not by purchasing an expensive twenty-class package from a boutique fitness studio that you don't actually enjoy. Nor is it thinking that you have to consume alkaline water with fresh squeezed lemon. It's about starting small with attainable health behaviors. Note that I am very specifically using the term *health behaviors* and not *weight loss* because many methods that people use for weight loss aren't sustainable or healthy, and are disordered. This leads to inevitable regain of weight, weight cycling, and stress on the body and mind.

Specifically, "health behaviors are actions taken by individuals that affect health or mortality."[7] Examples of health behaviors can be quitting smoking and substance use, modifying eating patterns, drinking more water, increasing physical activity, getting more sleep, and adhering to prescribed medical treatments. And, more importantly, health behaviors are often discussed on an individual level, but they can be measured for groups and populations as well. So while the diet app on your phone is having you log in and track calories and categorize them into fun colors, that actually isn't modifying a health behavior. For example, we can all eat a copious number of cookies and lose weight for a bit if we stick to the calories-in-and-calories-out method. Why? Because we can eat within a certain calorie range. Many diets and apps operate on the 3,500 calories = 1 pound logic. As long as you're reducing your intake by 3,500 calories, you can easily drop a pound. Simple, right? I remember following this logic many times myself when I was still entrenched in diet culture. I logged my calories daily, down to the tiniest morsel, in the hopes of shedding weight. I'm not even exaggerating when I say that if I had eaten just half of one grape, I would Google the calories and then deduct half. For a grape. But I also would restrict myself so much that when I was craving Ben & Jerry's (which was always, since I forbade myself from eating it), I wouldn't eat most of the day and then would finish an entire pint in one sitting. Was this in my daily 1,400 calorie range? Yes. Would I consider this to be the healthiest action now? Absolutely not. But that's the thing: diet culture as a whole doesn't care how you get to your weight loss as long as you get there. It follows calories in and calories out (which is also an antiquated method, since we know the human body is more complex than a math equation). As far as the 3,500-calories rule, there is increasing evidence that it is antiquated. We now know that how our bodies burn calories depends on numerous factors, such as the type of food eaten, our body's metabolism, and our gut microbiome.[8] So, yes, you can eat the exact same number of calories as someone else yet have very different outcomes when it comes to weight. You know, good ol' body diversity.

So, for someone who thinks that weight loss is the solution to diabetes, would eating endless cookies within a certain calorie range work? Maybe for weight loss for a short period of time. But would that help us with blood sugar control? Not really, because again, weight isn't a behavior. And by the way, cookies are delicious and there are indeed ways to enjoy them even while managing blood sugar. Wink wink.

• THE SOCIAL DETERMINANTS OF HEALTH •

I mentioned above that we sometimes equate health with thinness. And it really makes sense because we are constantly being told that having a higher weight is related to all sorts of health issues. This is why those in larger bodies are given the blanket advice of weight loss. But often, the actions that are taken toward weight loss aren't healthy. Ask yourself the following:

- Is it healthy to restrict our food intake to the point of constantly thinking about food and then telling ourselves we are obsessed with food?

- Is it healthy to let stress affect us both mentally and physically?

- Is it healthy to exercise to the point of injury and burn-out to just burn calories?

- Is it healthy to disengage and withdraw from social events and connections because of the fear around food and the inability to "control" ourselves around food?

How can we really define intentional weight loss as the epitome of health? To be hyperfixated on shrinking ourselves at the expense of our mental and physical well-being is the opposite of health. I say all these things not only from what I see with clients but also from experience. I have resided in what would be a socially accepted thin body, and I emphasize this because despite personal feelings, I have never been told or encouraged to lose weight while at the doctor. I never have issues going shopping for clothes because I know I will find my size at most stores. I fit into airplane seats and other "standard" seating. Despite what other ways we might be marginalized (I am Black and also a woman), we have to acknowledge the privileges we do have (I have a thin body, am cisgender, educated, and nondisabled) even when they seem to cancel each other out (I am discriminated against because of my race and gender daily and carry generational trauma because of the racial history within this country). And yet despite all my privileges, I was also susceptible to diet culture. My obsessive calorie tracking and overexercising was taking a toll, which I didn't realize at the time. Even when I stopped menstruating. Even when my hair was thinning. Even when I missed my friend's birthday celebration because I "couldn't" miss my dance class, since I needed to make up for the food I had eaten during the week.

Yes, I actually declined a friend's celebration because I was legitimately afraid of my body deteriorating from missing one day of class and eating some cake. Seriously. Does this sound healthy? There might be some people who are still trapped in the world of disordered eating who might commend this behavior as having willpower and taking accountability. But I know better now. Having strong social connections is one of the many health behaviors we can have. This might sound surprising because we always assume that just eating and exercising are the only healthy habits to improve upon, but this is far from the truth. While missing a single party isn't detrimental to health, when we are in a state where we feel the need to obsessively control ourselves, it is never a one-off event.

As humans, we are wired to connect and be social, which affects our health. Social support and feeling connected can help people control blood sugars, increase the odds of cancer survival, decrease cardiovascular mortality, decrease depressive symptoms, lessen post-traumatic stress disorder symptoms, and improve overall mental health. Social isolation, on the other hand, has a negative effect on our health and can increase depressive symptoms as well as mortality.[9] This is why it's so important to acknowledge health behaviors as a whole. We are conditioned to view eating and exercising as what determines our health and also our body size, but there is so much more. In fact, if we look at a pie chart, how we eat and how we move are mere slivers of what contributes to our health.

There are so many contributing health factors that are outside our control as individuals. According to the CDC, social determinants of health (SDOH) are the conditions in the environments where people are born, live, learn, work, play, worship, and age that affect a wide range of health, functioning, and quality of life outcomes and risks.[10]

Social Determinants of Health

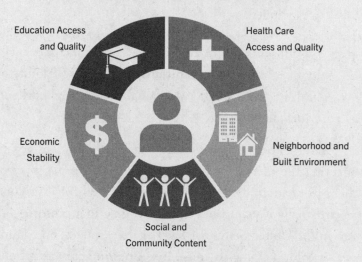

"*Social Determinants of Health,*" *Healthy People 2030, US Department of Health and Human Services, n.d., https://health.gov/healthypeople /priority-areas/social-determinants-health.*

SDOH can be divided into five categories:

- Health care access and quality: This can include equitable access to nonbiased health care, health insurance coverage, and literacy.

- Education access and quality: This can include equitable access to quality health care, enrollment in higher education, language and literacy, and childhood education and development.

- Social community: The characteristics of where people live, learn, work, and play.

- Economic stability: Financial resources, including income, cost of living, and socioeconomic status. Poverty, employment, food security, and housing stability are included.

- Neighborhood and environment: This includes quality of housing, access to transportation, availability of healthy foods, air and water quality, and neighborhood crime and violence.[11]

Also, it's notable that the CDC has cited racism as negatively affecting the mental and physical health of people, preventing them from attaining their highest level of health.[12] As a country, we are finally realizing and acknowledging that centuries of racism in the United States has had negative impacts on communities of color, helping to create inequities in access to a range of social and economic benefits such as housing, education, wealth, and employment. These are all included in the social determinants of health. These health inequities within communities of color place members of these populations at greater risk for poor health outcomes. I make note of this because we often rattle off statistics of higher rates of illness and death (including diabetes, hypertension, "obesity," asthma, and heart disease) among certain populations, especially when compared to white counterparts. Additionally, the life expectancy of non-Hispanic Black Americans is four years lower than that of white Americans.

Health is not something that is easily controllable by the individual. We get so caught up in thinking of ways to shrink ourselves and control every morsel of food that we put in our bodies that we forget about the external determinants and factors that have an effect on us. So, I ask, what if we focused on actual health behaviors instead of a solely physical transformation? Thinness does not equate to health because bodies are not business cards. When you look at a business card, you only see select information about an individual. It doesn't represent the individual's full identity. We look at someone's physical body the same way and judge their health status on what they look like and, based on that look, treat them accordingly. We live in a society that highly values an unrealistic ideal for everyone (thin, able-bodied, cisgender, Eurocentric), so I understand why it's tough to separate the pursuit of health from the pursuit of thinness. We sacrifice our physical and mental health in pursuit of thinness, which is completely contradictory to the fact that we say our actions *are* for improving our health. If we were truly discussing health, we would also discuss better sleep, adding nourishing foods, reducing stress, working on mental health, improving stamina and flexibility with exercise, and building social connections, which all actually correlate to health. But we look at bodies as business cards and think that our health is improving solely based on our bodies shrinking. That's why before and after pictures are so popular; it's a way to show how "healthy" an individual has become. But has the health of that individual actually improved, or did they just get thin? It's hard and maybe not as sexy to show a graph of improved sleeping habits or a decrease in mental health. If there's no before and after pic, then none of the improved health habits count, right? Even if you are finding that you have more energy and better mental clarity with improved sleep, it will still not be praised in the way weight loss is.

The bottom line is to always ask whether whatever method

you go about in pursuing health is in fact sustainable. Going on diets is like running on a hamster wheel. It's endless and it leaves you going through a cycle where you end up back at the beginning. It lures you in with false promises and the idea that you somehow lack willpower and control when the diet fails. It's a multibillion-dollar industry, so it depends on your failure. It doesn't matter that we all have different genetics, socioeconomic statuses, access, and more. We all have different bodies, so health will look different for all of us.

CHAPTER THREE

WE CANNOT BE CARBON COPIES OF EACH OTHER

Since I don't look like every other girl, it takes a while to be okay with that. To be different. But different is good.
—Serena Williams[1]

Before we move forward, an important **trigger warning**. This chapter will use language that some might find harmful and triggering—the dreaded *o* words: "obese," "obesity," and "overweight." Why is this harmful? Obese comes from the Latin *obesus*, which means "having eaten oneself fat,"[2] a phrasing that many fat activists classify as dehumanizing because, well, it is. I use the word *fat* because it is a description of a body (like thin), and therefore it should not have a negative connotation. I fully understand that this may be triggering, especially coming from someone in a thin body. Please note that I make it a point to actively learn from self-identifying fat activists and acknowledge that not everyone shares these views.

I'm not a gambling woman, but one thing I am 100 percent willing to put money on is the fact that there will always be some version of an influencer out there advertising a contorting body program. They will use words such as *transform*, *tone*, *lengthen*, and *sculpt*. They will show themselves performing certain exercises while simultaneously talking about how refreshed and rejuvenated they feel. They will have people who have partaken in these routines show photos of befores and afters. We are so used to seeing these images that we are desensitized to the subtle but blatant messaging that is there. Exercise has many great benefits, but talking about how it can improve brain health, reduce the risk of disease, strengthen bones and muscles, and improve your ability to do everyday tasks[3] just isn't as sexy as weight loss. Perfectly curated images sell. Talking about how you are now able to sit up straighter isn't as eye-catching as someone flashing their six-pack. We like to see images, and we like to see proof of effort.

But we cannot all look the same. We have different genetic makeups, so not everyone will have these advertised physical results, no matter how many lunges they do. So, what happens if you see that you don't look like that influencer? Even if you feel better, you think that you failed because you aren't transforming physically. We compare ourselves to people we see even though we aren't aware of the full picture. Genetics are, of course, at play, but there might also be disordered eating and other habits we can't see when looking at a person.

Genetics cause our bodies to come in all different shades, colors, and lengths, but for some reason we tend to think we should all be one size, some version of thin. It's like going to choose a paint color and only selecting colors like hale navy, ultrablue, and laguna. They are all a bit different, but they are all still shades of blue. Plus, many people assume if it isn't genetic, then working hard and eating a certain way can make us all thin. But the truth is there are multiple factors that influence our weight. Family history, family habits, culture, racial background, age, sex, medications, mental health, and the environment where we live, work, and worship all play a role.[4]

Further, we aren't supposed to look the same throughout our lifetime, no matter what influencer is trying to convince you to do a fit-into-your-high-school-jeans challenge. We often see celebrities being praised for looking the same or maintaining their physique with age. We are often bombarded with headlines such as "16 Ways Jennifer Lopez Makes 51 Look 31"[5] and "Jennifer Lopez's Rules for Ageless Beauty."[6] Should we take this to mean that at age fifty we should have the same physique and vitality as we did when we were twenty-five? (In case it wasn't clear: no!) And I know that J.Lo and other celebrities work hard for their bodies, but if we need to exercise multiple times a day to maintain a certain aesthetic, that's not a natural aesthetic. I empathize with the difficulties of being in the spotlight, but that doesn't make someone an expert on health. It also doesn't mean that we are doing something wrong if we notice our own bodies change.

We also must remember that what we are seeing in the media is not always reality thanks to filters, Facetuning, and editing. Plus, the type of lifestyle these celebrities have isn't accessible for all of us. Much of the pressure we feel is due to the societal narrative that we should all be some version of thin. Science backs this up. A study from the journal *Body Image* surveyed 227 female college students and found that "young women who spend more time on Facebook may feel more concerned about their body because they compare their appearance to others."[7]

Despite our seeming aversion to it, body diversity is nothing new. Past civilizations saw excess body fat as a symbol of wealth and prosperity as the general population struggled with food shortages and famine.[8] Roughly between 1500 and 1900, larger bodies, for both men and women, were preferred visually. There were variations according to country and century, but in general it was considered not only beautiful but natural to look "physically substantial." In many art pieces, there was a wide range of people, from courtiers to servants and rural laborers, who were depicted as solidly fleshy and taking up a good deal of space.[9]

One of my favorite resources for a historical look at how bodies trended throughout the years is *Fearing the Black Body: The Racial Origins of Fat Phobia*, by Dr. Sabrina Strings, who currently teaches at the University of California, Irvine. I find when I post on the origins of diet culture, I receive comments from many who are often surprised at the direct connections between racism, white patriarchy, and fatphobia. We are often quick to point out that diets affect women, and that our patriarchal society wants women to be smaller. However, there is a hesitancy by white audiences to acknowledge the correlation with white supremacy because that would mean a responsibility on their part to dismantle white supremacy. This is all the more reason why Strings's work is so important to read, and I often recommend it as the stepping stone for anything related to body image.

Fatphobia, especially when referring to Black women, did not originate with medical findings but with the Enlightenment-era belief that fatness was evidence of "savagery" and racial inferiority. There was a need of evidence to explain the inferiority of Black women, so equating fatness with being lazy and unintelligent became a theme that has held on tight to this day, as we demonize fatness and equate it with inferior morality. I highly recommend Strings's book for a more detailed look into this history.

• THE RACIST ROOTS OF . . . •

Let's cut to the chase: BMI (body mass index) is one of the most problematic diagnostic tools there is. That doesn't stop it from being widely used. BMI is a common metric for defining anthropometric height/weight characteristics in adults and for classifying (categorizing) them into groups of "underweight, normal weight, overweight, and sublevels of obese."[10] Many members of the health care industry believe that BMI is a good measure of an individual's fatness and risk factors for many chronic diseases and illnesses, but the metric is incredibly flawed.

BMI was actually created by a Belgian mathematician and astronomer named Lambert Adolphe Jacques Quetelet in the 1800s. Yes, the 1800s. Quetelet's goal was to find and formulate *l'homme moyen* (the average man); he believed that the average value of body distribution should be an important concern in the study of human attributes.[11] Quetelet wrote in 1842, "If the average man were completely determined, we might, as I have already observed, consider him as the type of perfection; and everything differing from his proportions or condition, would constitute deformity and disease; everything found dissimilar, not only as regarded proportion and form, but as exceeding the observed limits, would constitute a monstrosity."[12] Hard pass.

It's not lost on me how setting out to discern the average man was a way to weed out the others (women, people of color, disabled, poor). Simply put, it's eugenics. And if eugenics isn't enough to dismiss BMI entirely, we should also acknowledge that BMI was intended to measure the health and weight of a population, not an individual. We are still using measurements that were based only on white men from the 1800s. And we know that it's antiquated. The CDC website has a page on BMI but has the following statement: "BMI can be used to screen for weight categories that may lead to health problems, but it is not diagnostic of the body fatness or health of an individual."[13]

BMI disregards factors such as age, sex, race, and bone density and can't differentiate between muscle and fat or actual lifestyle factors. It overestimates "obesity" in African Americans[14] and underestimates health risks in Asians.[15] Interestingly, however, the health risks associated with "obesity" are also influenced by race, with Black individuals at lower health risk and Asians at higher risk compared with whites at the same BMI. It's a flawed system, one that is used to discriminate. Some insurance companies might try to refuse coverage or make the rate higher for larger-weight individuals.[16] In 1998 the US National Institutes of Health brought US definitions in line with World Health Organization guidelines, lowering the normal/overweight cutoff from a BMI of 27.8 (men) and 27.3 (women) to a BMI of 25 for both sexes. As soon as these guidelines changed, CNN wrote in an article titled "Who's Fat? New Definition Adopted," "Some health experts reject the new guidelines, claiming people who aren't fat are now considered overweight. For example, under the new definitions, many professional athletes would be considered too heavy. Critics also worry that these lower weights will persuade doctors to start prescribing diet drugs for people who don't need them. Some diet drugs carry health risks, such as an increase in blood pressure."[17]

It doesn't stop there—for many eating disorder centers, insurers will use BMI to make coverage decisions and can limit treatment to those who qualify as underweight, dismissing a large number of others who need treatment. We are driven by numbers, which prevent many from getting the help they need. For example, atypical anorexia describes individuals who meet all of the criteria for anorexia nervosa except significant weight loss; the individual's weight is within or above the normal range.[18]

Here are some facts regarding atypical anorexia nervosa:

- Atypical anorexia nervosa hospitalizations make up nearly one-third of hospital inpatient eating disorder treatment programs.

- At least 40 percent of those struggling with atypical anorexia nervosa require admission to a hospital.

- Psychological distress related to eating and body image is worse in atypical anorexia than anorexia nervosa.[19]

It sounds radical, but there are ways to look at health without looking at weight or at BMI. Health is different for everyone and looks different for everyone. Health is also not a moral virtue. Due to genetics and the social determinants of health, there are many individuals who will never live up to society's version of health. This doesn't make someone less deserving of respect. Using an outdated formula as an excuse to discriminate against individuals is actually the opposite of helping.

Certain demographics also have a higher percentage of larger bodies than others. Being discriminated against because of size and because of race or other marginalized identities adds on many layers of trauma, which in turn can contribute to chronic diseases. Without a doubt, weight stigma has a detrimental effect on health. In health care settings, it can look like symptoms not being taken seriously because of a person's weight.

• WEIGHT STIGMA •

A. Janet Tomiyama, a professor of psychology at the University of California, Los Angeles, defines weight stigma, also known as weight bias or weight-based discrimination, as the social rejection and devaluation that accrues to those who do not comply with prevailing social norms of adequate body weight and shape.[20]

Weight stigma can increase body dissatisfaction, a leading risk factor in the development of eating disorders. Let's be super clear here: it is never acceptable to discriminate against someone based on their size, but shaming, blaming, and concern trolling happen everywhere—at work, at school, in the home, and even at the doctor's office. In fact, weight discrimination occurs more frequently than gender or age discrimination.

One study of primary care physicians found that more than 50 percent viewed "obese" patients as awkward, unattractive, and noncompliant. More than one-third of these physicians characterized "obese" patients as weak-willed, sloppy, and lazy. In another study, 45 percent of a sample of physicians agreed that they have a negative reaction to these individuals. Another study of military family physicians found that physicians' stereotypical views of finding these individuals lazy increased 145 percent between 1998 and 2005, with younger physicians more likely to endorse this attitude.[21]

Reviewing these statistics, it shouldn't be a surprise that many fat patients avoid seeking medical care. If a patient is receiving the message that they are unwelcome or devalued in a clinical setting and feel ignored and mistreated, they are less likely to go. Not to mention that those with a higher BMI are nearly three times as likely as persons with "normal" BMI to say they have been denied appropriate medical care.[22] Medical professionals themselves are not immune to experiencing weight bias. Medical students with a higher BMI report that clinical work can be particularly challenging, and those with a higher BMI who internalize anti-fat attitudes also report more depressive symptoms and alcohol or substance abuse.[23]

It bears repeating that weight stigma is dangerous. It can increase the risk for adverse psychological and behavioral issues, including depression, poor body image, and binge eating. And weight stigma also poses a significant threat to psychological and physical health. It is a risk factor for depression, body dissatisfaction, and low self-esteem. Those who experience weight-based stigmatization also

- Engage in more frequent binge eating;

- Are at an increased risk for eating disorder symptoms; and

- Are more likely to have a diagnosis for binge eating disorder (BED).[24]

What does weight stigma sound like from actual humans who experience it? I wrote an Instagram post on the subject in 2020, and I received some comments from those who were willing to tell their stories (comments taken from my actual Instagram post with the names removed):

One patient I was treating for neck pain had previously been told by another doc the pain would improve if weight was lost. NECK PAIN! I was so angry that I couldn't hide my emotions. How the hell can neck pain be caused by being fat?

That the clients sent to me to "lose weight" prior to conceiving isn't the problem. The REAL problem is doctors not doing thorough evals and listening to their patients!

In January I was severely anemic due to extreme bleeding. A hospital refused to treat me. They told me the bleeding was caused.. by my diet. I went to another hospital; it was eight cantaloupe-size fibroids. Eight!

So crazy that you shared this because I went to see my doctor for constant aches/pains and chills. I was told losing weight is the answer to my issues lol. I understand but also I've been "bigger" my entire life and I've never experienced chills or aches like this.

Unfortunately, these stories aren't surprising, because there is widespread weight bias in the medical field. Health care professionals are told of the "obesity epidemic" that is plaguing society, but rarely discussed are the social and environmental factors that can affect health; the lack of acceptance of body diversity, which drives diet cycling, which contributes to weight cycling, which affects weight; and the way in which fat bodies are unwelcome in society. One of the biggest forms of stigma is biased health care, but stigma also comes in the form of individuals not having equal access to basic human necessities.

• LACK OF INCLUSIVITY •

My stint in fashion gave me an insider's understanding of the industry and how absurd it is that many brands and stores aren't size inclusive.

Sixty-eight percent of American women wear a size 14 or

above.[25] There is a market available for those sizes, but they are not as accessible as they should be. Experts in the industry will list a lack of distribution, store size, and qualities as reasons why many stores don't carry more inclusive sizes; however, it still doesn't make sense given the demographic of more than two-thirds of American women in need of more inclusive sizes.[26] And appropriate clothing choices aren't just wants—they're necessities. In Article 25 of the United Nations' Universal Declaration of Human Rights, clothing is listed as a standard of living for adequate health and well-being, along with food and housing.[27]

Fashion isn't the only area that lacks inclusion. Seating size is also a major problem. A content creator shared on social media that she couldn't fit on the roller coaster at Universal Studios. She mentioned that not only was the space not accommodating but she was also humiliated because she was forced to test out the seats in front of other visitors and her children.[28] She shared that even though she is active and healthy, she still couldn't enjoy a day with her family due to this humiliation. This particular story went viral on TikTok mostly because her story resonated with so many. So many folks shared humiliating stories of not being able to fit into airplane seats or theater seats at movies and concerts, having ill-fitting equipment at doctors' offices, and much more. The world doesn't have to tell you with words that you are unwelcome—it can easily show you.

Since the 1990s, the width of airplane seats has shrunk from 18 inches to about 16 inches, and the distance between seat backs has decreased from 35 inches to sometimes less than 28 inches.[29] That is incredibly uncomfortable for many folks, but it is especially concerning when the average man in the US has a 40.5-inch waist and the average female a 38.7-inch waist.[30] As

Aubrey Gordon, fat activist and author of *What We Don't Talk About When We Talk about Fat*, writes, "Our cultural conversations about flying while fat also reinforce anti-fat judgment. We talk about fat passengers with scorn, insisting that if they don't like it, they can just lose weight. In so doing, we imply that fat people are responsible for the discriminatory policies, not the airlines who wrote them."[31]

It's sort of mind-boggling (but not surprising) that we spend our time worried about the degree of someone's health based on what their physical body looks like, rather than providing them with basic human needs. Society tells people in larger bodies to get healthy but at the same time creates a toxic environment that ostracizes and excludes them. Instead of accepting diverse shapes and sizes, we create an environment where everyone is made to feel that they should assimilate and conform. It takes more than body positivity and daily affirmations to stand up to systemic barriers; it takes actual liberation.

• FAT LIBERATION •

Body positivity is the general idea that all bodies are good bodies, and today's body positivity movement would be nothing without fat liberation. Fat activism started in the 1960s at the same time the women's liberation movement and Black civil rights were gaining momentum. The movement originated from fat, Black, and queer activism that was organized in response to certain bodies being so rarely visible or held as valuable in discourses and visual media.[32] Fat activists saw fat liberation linked to other struggles of oppression, such as racism and LGBTQ+ rights. In 1969, the National Association to Aid Fat Americans (now called the National Association to Advance Fat Acceptance, or NAAFA) was created in response to the discrimination people in larger bodies face.[33]

In 1972, activist Johnnie Tillmon said, "I'm a woman. I'm a Black woman. I'm a poor woman. I'm a fat woman. I'm a middle-aged woman. In this country, if you're any one of those things, you count less as a human being."[34] That statement perfectly encapsulated the heart of the movement. Black women were often labeled fat, ugly, and sluggish in the media. This fueled the movement to focus on fatphobia as the product of misogyny and racism.

Even with the strong origins of this movement, it seems that somewhere along the way it took a sharp detour and derailed. When you look at images on social media, the majority of "positive" bodies you see are young, white, lean, able-bodied, and cis women. The movement quite often lacks discussion around intersectionality. It's hard to discuss how all bodies are good bodies when society still tells us that the only good bodies are the more socially accepted thin ones. There is more and more pushback by fat activists against using the term *body positivity* because in order to actually promote the statement that all bodies are good bodies, the most marginalized of those bodies should be front and center. We have to center those voices. I have stopped using the term *body positivity* on my posts as well because it doesn't describe the real disruption I want for the system. I want actual body diversity to be celebrated and normalized.

The original purpose of the body positivity movement was to highlight discrimination and fatphobia that larger-bodied people faced, but the general tenor of it has lost its purpose. We are all allowed to have off days with our bodies, but there is a difference between your body being policed and discriminated against and having an off day. Body positivity preaches "love your body no matter what," which is helpful for some. However, fat activism takes us deeper (to body positivity's original roots) and says "my body is not a disease, and I deserve equitable treatment and to not be discriminated against." There's a difference.

If you want to learn about racism, especially anti-Blackness, you should learn it from someone Black. If you want to learn about discrimination that the LGBTQ+ community faces, you should learn it from someone who is part of the LGBTQ+ community. If you want to learn about weight stigma and bias and the harm they perpetuate, you need to learn from a fat activist. I say this intentionally because I don't want to be someone's sole or main source regarding anti-fatness and weight stigma. We need to be more intentional about learning from lived experiences. This is why there should never be an event about weight stigma with no fat folks. The same way in which a panel on anti-Blackness having no Black folks would, and should, cause an uproar, a panel on weight stigma with no fat people should have the same effect.

Social media can be a place for learning, but it can also make us feel as though we are in a bubble. If we are not actively looking for certain content or creators, we are shown only one type of physicality and/or ideas. This can be due in part to the algorithm that pushes out certain content while suppressing others, but we also tend to feel more comfortable with seeing people who look like us or bodies we are socialized to uphold. I always recommend diversifying your feed for this exact reason.

The body positivity movement we see today looks drastically different from its origins because we still privilege thin bodies. Body positivity tells people that they are allowed to have doubts and love their imperfections, as long as they are still a version of thin and conventionally attractive. How would we know that there are many versions of bodies, and that body diversity is actually normal, if we are only living and existing in our bubble and not intentionally seeking out people who are diverse? We tend to seek out and follow people who look like us on social media, and even if those people don't look like us per se, they represent an image that we would want to attain or find desirable. I think back to June 2020 when #BlackoutTuesday was running rampant in response to the racial tension due to the murder of George Floyd. Many social media accounts proudly put up a black square as a way to show solidarity, but it didn't stop there. So many non-Black social media users realized they didn't follow any Black accounts and flocked to try to find and follow as many as they could. This had positive and negative effects. On a positive note, so many accounts (including mine) were being recognized and acknowledged as learning tools by folks who otherwise would not seek out our work. On a negative note, many of these acts of solidarity were performative. But we shouldn't have to wait for a movement to realize that our feed and the people we seek education from only look one way. Diversity in every aspect should be something that we look for and want to change with intention.

This doesn't happen overnight. We must sit with discomfort and acknowledge that the information we had for many years might not have been entirely correct. We can accept that diet culture is not doing anything helpful for society, but we have trouble accepting body diversity and that some bodies are fat. Many social media posts will say things like "I'm all for body positivity, but" or "People shouldn't be discriminated against, but." There shouldn't be any buts after any statement.

I am not denying someone's lived experience in any capacity. Many folks say they feel better with weight loss. I believe them. I believe them because I imagine it feels better when you are being treated more positively by conforming instead of constantly fighting with society. I imagine it feels better to find clothes more easily and to fit in seating areas. I'm not denying that. I'm also not denying that joints feel better, and you have more energy with weight loss because maybe you are receiving proper physical therapy and feel more welcome in public exercise spaces. I imagine that there was a change with behavior and that maybe it might be doing exercises that are actually strengthening your muscles and increasing your stamina. It might not just be weight loss and having a smaller body. I say might, because I am not denying anyone's experience or telling someone how to feel. Body autonomy is incredibly important, but so is body acceptance.

Further Reading

Stephanie Yeboah, *Fattily Ever After: A Black Fat Girl's Guide to Living Life Unapologetically*[35]

Da'Shaun L. Harrison, *Belly of the Beast: The Politics of Anti-Fatness as Anti-Blackness*[36]

Sonya Renee Taylor, *The Body Is Not an Apology: The Power of Radical Self-Love*[37]

Roxane Gay, *Hunger: A Memoir of (My) Body*[38]

Aubrey Gordon, *What We Don't Talk About When We Talk About Fat*[39]

Dr. Sabrina Strings, *Fearing the Black Body: The Racial Origins of Fat Phobia*[40]

· CHAPTER FOUR ·

ELITISM OF HEALTH AND WELLNESS

Over 450 million Indians live under the poverty line, yet
wellness—particularly yoga—is a multibillion-dollar industry
extracted from our culture.
—Fariha Róisín[1]

• LET'S GET SOME THINGS STRAIGHT •

What really is wellness? Is it a yoga retreat at a bungalow in Costa
Rica? Is it blue spirulina that you can put in your smoothie?
Is it a seventy-five-dollar candle that smells like Gwyneth Pal-
trow's vagina? (Hint: it's definitely not that). Frankly, the definition of wellness can vary drastically depending on who you
ask. The National Wellness Institute, an organization with the
goal of driving inclusive and optimal wellness for everyone
within their environment, defines wellness as "an active process through which people become aware of, and make choices
toward, a more successful existence."[2] But this leads to more
questions, like how do we define a "more successful existence"?
The openness of that phrase makes it sound like wellness could
include a multitude of different things, including career choices
or dating modes or being a good parent, but that's not the successful existence wellness is referring to; instead, wellness is

often used as a synonym for health, and trust me, they are not the same thing.

Wellness and diet culture often go hand in hand. They both stem from a place of desired perfection. From a young age, we are taught to think that if we have access to certain products and a certain lifestyle, we will have optimal health. The idea of wellness plays on our desire to show that if we try hard enough and spend enough money, if we can go above and beyond, we can be exceptional in terms of health. Because it is intertwined with diet culture, wellness therefore is rooted in the desire to obtain a thin, Eurocentric ideal at all costs. This in turn can lead to a wide variety of negative outcomes, including causing non-Eurocentric identities to feel the need to conform or alter their cultural dishes. Many cultures are told their food is not good enough. Their bodies are not good enough. They are not good enough.

And just so we're clear here, wellness is not the same as being healthy. According to the World Health Organization (WHO), health is a state of complete physical, mental, and social well-being and not merely the absence of disease or infirmity.[3] Let me point out that each individual's health is unique and therefore different. We can aspire to physical health, meaning increasing activity to maintain and/or strengthen our bones, muscles, and joints. We can aspire to mental health by working on our stress levels. For our social well-being, we can try to balance our social and personal lives. These measures fall under the scope of health, and health serves as a currency in society, but not for the reasons one might think. Health is often associated with morality, and we uphold individuals who seem as though they are doing everything in their power to be as healthy as possible. So many people feel the need to prove their health status. That may look like constantly posting gym selfies or the healthy foods they're eating daily. We congratulate such individuals on making health a priority even though we don't know if they're exercising unsafely or excessively. We don't know about the exact foods someone is eating or if they are eating enough or practicing disordered habits. But we don't seem to care about those details because we see a thin body or someone who is actively working toward a thin body. Thanks to diet culture, we say that we uphold and care about health, but we are really upholding beauty standards. The only reason we care about what someone is or isn't doing is because of what they look like.

Wellness aims to *enhance* our health status. So that SoulCycle class is enhancing your physical health. Going on a yoga retreat might be enhancing your physical and mental health. And I guess somewhere in this spectrum, a seventy-five-dollar vagina candle could also be described as enhancing. But wellness and health are inextricably entwined in our minds, making the idea of health, an age-old concept that simply means soundness of body and mind, something of a hot topic. With the onset of wellness, we've made health into a kind of status symbol, a way of keeping up with the Joneses (or the Kardashians). Wellness is targeted to a group of individuals who are looking beyond mainstream Western medicine and beyond mainstream health.

Now, don't get me wrong—I love some bougie things just as much as the next person. I was a SoulCycle fanatic years ago, riding and tapping it back in a dark room with a modelesque instructor at 6:00 a.m. I love those overpriced fifteen-dollar green fresh-pressed juices because they are indeed refreshing and tasty. So really, this is not a knock on anyone who participates in wellness culture.

But in actuality, are certain foods and products really superior for your health, or are they just appealing because they're expensive and not easily accessible for everyone? Because here's the thing: wellness attracts the elite, and it can be so easy to fall into the idea of wanting to be a part of this exclusive club. And it is indeed selective: for example, in 2021, tickets for In Goop Health, a health and wellness summit, had a one-thousand-dollar starting price.[4] When it comes to wellness, the fact that it is not readily available to the masses seems to heighten its appeal. After all, why would you want something everyone can afford? If anyone can afford a protein powder, is it really exclusive? Could the product still be considered superior?

If anyone can afford it, it's not as attractive for many, and that's just part of how the wellness industry operates. Wellness is like that exclusive club in New York City or Miami where you see a line out the door and everyone in that line looks like a model. You don't even know what's going on inside, but all those incredibly cool people want in, so it must be great, right? Some people are being let in and others are being turned away, which makes it more enticing. You want that elite access, too. But when the bouncer finally lets you in, it turns out there's actually nothing all that special going on in there, and the drinks and the food are overpriced. Like that protein powder that anyone can buy is pretty much exactly the same as the one sold exclusively by a wellness influencer—but it doesn't come in as pretty a package or with as cool a name.

So why do influencers and ads keep on pushing these "exclusive" products? Because there is some serious money to be made there. The global wellness market has an estimated worth of more than $1.5 trillion. This goes well beyond eating fruits and vegetables. More than a third of consumers around the world report that they "probably" or "definitely" plan to increase spending on nutrition apps, diet programs, juice cleanses, and subscription food services over the next year.[5] The laws of supply and demand apply in the wellness industry just as they do everywhere else. You start with a want; you raise the price, thus making the product more elusive; and eventually the want becomes a need. Throw in a couple of influencers and celebrities claiming the magic formula works, and you've got yourself a sought-after product. Add all those products together, and you've got yourself an expensive and exclusive lifestyle.

We should remember that on social media, not everything is what it seems. Social media is, in a way, the presentation of fantasy. We like to peek into other people's lives and see how they are traveling, eating, exercising, and living. Many of us are visual creatures and like to look at aesthetically pretty pictures and videos. This is why there are so many filters available and why so many people feel like they have to look a certain way in order to be presentable. This is also why we can't always trust what we are seeing on social media because many people are carefully curating their feeds to give you an impression of them that's not totally accurate.

This can hold true for the way someone presents what they are eating. Most of the foods that are shown are nutrient-dense items that the influencer advertises and tells us they eat in order to look and feel the way they do. Even though many of these foods are nutrient dense, some of the habits and the way these foods are being eaten can be considered disordered. Skipping meals, cutting out food groups, exercising excessively, and compulsively checking labels are all examples.

Of course, we have a right to know what's in our food and if it contains ingredients that could be harmful. But we need to pay attention to how and where we are getting that information. We should be listening to food scientists and engineers who are knowledgeable and have studied and immersed themselves in these topics. But because so much content on social media is based on aesthetics and trends, it is often hard to find credible resources and content creators.

Many products and lifestyle changes that are popular are based upon putting certain foods in a hierarchy. We have our "good" foods that are given the halo of approval by folks in the wellness community and are usually described as "pure" or "natural." One way to describe this natural category is by dubbing it *clean*. Scrolling through social media, you constantly see posts about clean recipes, clean meals, clean foods. You get the idea. But in actuality, what does *clean* mean?

• CLEAN EATING •

One quick Google search demonstrates that there are many interpretations of what *clean* means in terms of eating and food. When I see examples of clean eating plans, there are some nourishing foods, yes, but it's hard to identify what makes them clean exactly. Meals that are composed of a variety of vegetables don't make a dish clean; the vegetables make it nutrient dense. I also constantly hear people say that they eat clean, and again I ask what does that mean? Some people will say eating more fruits and vegetables, and others will say eating organic. There's no specific answer, partially because *clean eating* is a term that doesn't really mean anything. It's just a label anyone can put on a recipe or product to make it more attractive to a consumer.

Clean food lists vary but usually include fruits, vegetables, whole grains, and lean proteins. Added sugars, sodium, and fat are big nos. There is nothing wrong with wanting to get in nutrients and eating a variety of foods, but there is something about defining the way we eat as clean that needs to be reexamined. If you say that you are eating clean, are other foods dirty? Food, unless it's covered in soot, isn't dirty, and using the word *clean* to describe food implies healthiest or purest, which is just another way to be elitist about food.

In my humble opinion, clean food means washing your produce before consumption and making sure you have a napkin handy when eating something messy. It can even mean following the ten-second rule and not eating what has dropped to the floor. It has different interpretations to us all.

When the International Food Information Council (IFIC) polled consumers in June 2021 on what they thought *clean* meant,

- 21 percent said eating foods that aren't highly processed,

- 14 percent said eating foods found in the fresh produce section,

- 13 percent said eating organic,

- 11 percent said eating foods with simple ingredient lists, and

- 9 percent said eating foods with ingredients they consider clean.[6]

You can eat what you want, of course, and different foods will work better for our individual bodies, but what the public needs to understand is that clean eating is just a buzzword. It's not specifically defined by any governing body or industry.

• THE HEALTHIFYING OF CULTURAL FOODS •

This elitism extends to the way we often try to "healthify," or clean up, different foods, many of which are cultural. Call it what you like, but this is just straight-up racism. In countless weight-loss programs, health retreats, and clean-eating cleanses, cultural staples are frequently removed and replaced with more Westernized and Eurocentric substitutes. For example, the substitution of cauliflower for rice (one of the many demon carbohydrates) is a common "love this cultural food, but not like this" message that runs rampant.

Whether we realize it or not, we tend to associate certain cultural foods with bad choices, or cheat meals. There are constant memes on social media correlating Mexican and Chinese dishes with cheat meals all the time—for instance, "If you had to choose between tacos and being skinny, are you choosing soft or hard tacos?" is one I come across a lot on Pinterest. Tacos are a cultural food, and demoting them to simply a cheat meal—in other words, a scheduled meal consisting of what's considered indulgent or unhealthy food—is extremely stigmatizing. Imagine a food that is prominent in your culture and has meaning within your family being referred to as something unhealthy that people should feel guilty about eating. Even if we ignore the actual nutrients of these foods—yeah, they're already healthy—it is wrong and harmful to ignore the familial traditions and heritage tied to these cuisines.

The need to healthify cultural cuisines sends the message that these cultures are inherently unhealthy and need to be fixed. For example, there are many cookbooks out on shelves that offer "healthier" versions of various cultural cuisines, written by people not of those cultures. You will see recipes that substitute ingredients such as different grains and oils in the name of health. This is all fine if someone wants to swap out ingredients on an individual level for their personal needs, but to call it a healthier recipe in general is not only culturally insensitive and stigmatizing, it is downright xenophobic. No matter what the intention, attempting to improve a culture's food, especially when you are not of that culture, is deeply problematic. And on the other side of this, so many cultural foods or traditions have been co-opted by mainstream wellness. In other words, cultural foods and traditions are often looked down upon and questioned, unless they can be rebranded and Westernized for profit. I'm talking about yoga, Ayurveda, dry brushing, bone broth, turmeric, avocados, chia seeds, and—trust me, I could go on and on.

The most disastrous result is that people of various ethnicities come to view themselves as unhealthy because of society's dismissal of the cultural staples of their diets. In academia, we learn that certain populations are more likely to have certain illnesses and diseases, and the cause is often ascribed to diet; stress factors like poverty and racism are almost never discussed. For example, at 14.5 percent, American Indians and Alaska Natives have the highest rates of diagnosed diabetes among any race or ethnicity.[7] In conjunction with this statistic, this population also has a higher amount of inequity in health care and health status compared to other US populations. Health outcomes are adversely affected by inadequate access to comprehensive health services. American Indians and Alaska Natives born today have a life expectancy that is 4.4 years less than all other races in the United States.[8] Even with the strong correlation between inequity and health, some medical professionals shake their heads, believing that these populations inherently don't care about their health and that diet is the reason why these populations have higher BMIs.

My nutrition courses consisted of classes that often discussed public health and noted that marginalized BIPOC populations were dealing with little access to health care, systemic racism, low income, weight stigmatization, misogyny, and dozens of other factors that contributed to these illnesses. However, it is always emphasized that people are in control of their own destiny and that with a few food tweaks their lives would automatically improve, and they have the power to do this themselves. Hardly anyone mentions that many of these populations have a deep distrust of the medical field as a whole because of its racist origins and therefore many do not choose to seek regular medical attention. Thinking back to my own schooling, we weren't given enough instruction on cultural competency or respecting the values, traditions, and beliefs of other cultures and to be aware of our own biases. There was always the assumption that someone doesn't care about their health or, because someone is of a certain culture, they only eat in one way. This isn't true, and society as a whole needs to be more aware of these thoughts. Imagine being told that your culture is unhealthy and that a dish that includes tortilla chips and guacamole is labeled a cheat meal, while at the same time being able to walk into any artisanal overpriced café and order avocado toast. The irony.

• THE WELLNESS INFLUENCERS •

With all the new wellness products and trends that permeate our lives, there will always be a need for their promotion to the public. Enter the influencer. Take a quick look at the top wellness influencers on social media and you'll see (mostly) cishet, white, thin, and nondisabled people roaming grocery store aisles and highlighting foods that "you should avoid" or making "here's what I eat in a day" reels. Seeing these influencers pop up on your social feeds can make it easy to forget that these are players in the wellness field, and that they have an agenda and a personal brand. Be as skeptical of them as you would of any corporation or public figure.

So before you start changing your habits based on what an influencer says, remember that they may be operating with the following business model in mind:

Step 1: They know their audience. People want to know what the secret to health is. It can't be as simple as fruits and vegetables. It must be something more extreme, something less obvious. Because the audience needs to ask, What's the secret? Influencers are betting that you'll want to know.

Step 2: Influencers then cater to the fears of the audience. So much of this messaging is capitalizing on the fact that many people distrust our food system. *The government is trying to poison us!* or *Companies are paying off the government in order to put whatever they want in our food.* These worries are especially powerful when it comes to parents who want to feed their children the very best. But the best isn't always what we think it is.

Step 3: Influencers use an authoritative, fearmongering voice. Messages like *Don't eat this product. It has high-fructose corn syrup and artificial colors that are banned in other countries. You could die.* Or *This preservative listed* *here is actually petroleum! They're putting petroleum in our food!* Okay, got it. With all this messaging, it's easy to see why people feel anxious or stressed around food choices.

Step 4: Influencers make their money. You think these people are warning us about these things from the goodness of their hearts? Ha! No way. If there are a bunch of things we *shouldn't* be eating, then that means there is a need for products we *should* be eating. And if not products, there is always a need for programs, lists of don'ts, YouTube channels, Instagram ads, etc. Because they're exclusive, these products can't be found in local supermarkets, aren't eligible for SNAP (Supplemental Nutrition Assistance Program) and EBT (Electronic Benefit Transfer), and aren't at an affordable price point. You have to get it straight from the influencer.

To be a wellness influencer, you don't need credentials or experience to state your opinions, no matter how incorrect, misinformed, or dangerous they may be. So, are all influencers problematic? No, absolutely not, and even the promotion of certain foods isn't automatically harmful. However, there is a direct correlation between many narratives shared by these folks and misinformation that is spread. The term *misinformation* refers to information that is false or inaccurate and often spread widely, regardless of an intent to deceive.[9] Misinformation doesn't just stop at food and what an influencer deems healthy and not healthy. Part of the appeal of wellness practitioners is the way they respond to people's unmet health and medical needs. Wellness culture has given rise to an industry of self-appointed lifestyle and wellness gurus who combine nutritional advice and exercise tips with self-development and new age spirituality. There is a specific theme here of taking responsibility for one's own health. It is apparently up to the individual to eat certain foods and practice certain methods that will promote their own longevity.

It's pretty easy now to promote beliefs and rhetoric with technology being conveniently at our fingertips. Social media is ubiquitous, and this is how many influencers are able to market themselves to the public. For example, the platform TikTok reported 1 billion active users as of 2021.[10] That's a huge amount of people and information being presented. With TikTok, users have quick access to someone they admire and watch their whole day unfold as if they were in the same room as this person. What is this person going to choose to wear? How are they going to do their makeup? What are they going to eat? If I eat like them, will I, too, look like them? This is the lane where the What I Eat in a Day (WIEIAD) videos thrive, and this trend is particularly problematic. Now, these are not just recipes or how-to videos. These videos are a "full" look into what influencers are eating. I put *full* in quotation marks because we never actually know whether what we're viewing is or isn't real. Only through videos do we see the meals and foods that the influencer is consuming. I must emphasize that these are not the same thing as being shown recipes or grocery hauls. The WIEIAD has the purpose of showing the good foods that are being consumed and, in a way, it is sort of an advertisement for how the influencer looks the way they do, because many also advertise their bodies as achievable end results. Let me remind you that eating like someone will not make you look like them.

We tend to look at someone and base their credibility solely on their appearance. So what we are likely to see on social media is the influencer who tells us to only eat organic. And just to get some things straight on what *organic* really means: Organic certification is regulated by the United States Department of Agriculture (USDA), which is, you know, a government agency. Organic certification allows a farm or processing facility to sell, label, and represent their products as organic. USDA-certified organic foods are grown and processed according to federal guidelines addressing, among many factors, soil quality, animal raising practices, pest and weed control, and use of additives.[11] That does not mean these farming practices don't use pesticides. Most importantly, it does not mean that the nutritional quality of the produce is superior—there is no evidence suggesting it is.

Let's also clear some things up about products from European countries and their "superiority." Quite often, ingredients labeled on their products look shorter and easier to read, but that does not mean they are superior in content. In the US, we use a risk-based approach to banning products, meaning we consider potential to cause harm, as well as the potential harm of exposure, when regulating products. Not many countries do this. The UK, for example, uses a hazard-based approach to regulation, meaning something that can *potentially* cause harm. Huh? This is confusing, right? In summary, hazard-based approaches (UK) use the presence of a potentially harmful agent at a detectable level in food in order to label it a risk. Risk-based approaches (US), on the other hand, allow consideration of exposure in determining whether there are risks to health. A hazard is an agent that has the potential to cause harm, while a risk measures the likelihood of harm from a hazard.

David Zaruk, founder of GreenFacts and an environmental-health risk governance analyst, states the following: "A hazard (like a car) is only a risk if we are involved in a crash or it hits us while moving."[12] In other words, a hazard like a car only becomes a danger (risk) when it can severely impact us. If someone does not expose themselves to moving cars in traffic, there is no risk. Said in more scientific terms: **Risk** takes into consideration the **Hazard** and the **Exposure** level to that **Hazard** (Risk = Hazard + Exposure).

Hazard

Something that can potentially cause harm

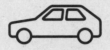

Risk

Assesses both the Hazard and the Exposure to the Hazard

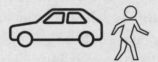

Food safety and its logistics are confusing to the everyday person who is not well versed in this field. This is all the more reason why we should listen to scientists on the matter, not Anna the influencer with the genetics and the curated pictures to look attractive, who is just reading the labels out loud. Erin, a food scientist and engineer of the social media account Food Science Babe, breaks this down perfectly. In an Instagram post, she points out the following:

> Formaldehyde can be hazardous to humans; however, our bodies produce it and we consume it in foods such as apples and pears. We know that at those doses it is not a

risk. Should we ban everything that contains formalde-hyde because it is a hazardous chemical? Of course not, but that's exactly the reasoning that's used when taking a hazard-based approach.[13]

Labeling regulations are also different among countries. In the US, we list spices and flavorings, while on the same product in the UK, you might just see "extract" and "spice." And as for those folks who go to Europe and claim to lose weight while there, let's just be clear that it's never just the food making you lose weight. It's also factors like a shift in work-life balance, being less sedentary while traveling, or a decrease in stress. When visiting Paris, are you viewing the Eiffel Tower and the Louvre while sitting statically, or is your body in a constant state of motion while visiting these historic sites? While vacationing in walkable cities, you are most likely moving, and that movement is probably more than you are used to in the US during your normal day-to-day life. It's nothing more revolutionary than that.

We think that European nations are healthier because of the food. In talking about that assumption, I always invite people to dig deeper and remember that many of those countries have completely different socioeconomic factors and lifestyles. We cannot compare apples to oranges. The United States might have more processed foods, but we should start to recognize the reasons why we need more processed foods. We should also recognize that processed foods are not inherently scary or problematic.

• WHAT ARE PROCESSED FOODS, ANYWAY? •

If allowed, people are intentional with their choices. According to the Food Industry Association, in 2021, 58 percent of shoppers were influenced by the healthfulness of a food product, and 43 percent said that it's important for a food/beverage to include only a few ingredients; and in 2020, 49 percent looked for minimal processing.[14] This isn't a surprise, given how popular headlines that discuss processed foods, how bad they are, and how to cut back and detox from them are. Nothing scares the wellness community more than the word *processed*, and you will usually see social media posts and headlines about how processed foods must be avoided at all costs.

But what is so terrifying about processed foods? The truth is that nearly everything we eat is processed to some degree, meaning that unless you go to an apple orchard and pick the apple from the tree and eat it right there, you are eating processed food. Processed simply means that the food has been manipulated in some way (which does not make it bad or unhealthy). This can include fruits and vegetables that were sprayed and packaged in preparation for travel to stores, bagged spinach and salads, and, of course, boxed and canned foods. The NOVA classification, which was developed by Brazilian nutrition researcher Carlos Monteiro, classifies foods into four groups according to their level of processing. The ranking and level of processing goes as follows:

- **Group 1:** Unprocessed or minimally processed foods, which include fresh and frozen fruits and vegetables, grains, meats, eggs, legumes, and nuts/seeds. Processing in this group means the removal of inedible parts and does not add substances to the original form.

- **Group 2:** Processed culinary ingredients, which include oils (olive, coconut, etc.), animal fats (butter), maple syrup, sugar, and honey. These are substances from group 1 foods that have been processed through pressing, refining, grinding, etc.

- **Group 3:** Processed foods, which include canned vegetables, fruit, meat, fish, cheese, bread, wine, beer, and cider. The processing in this group includes foods from groups 1 or 2 with the addition of oil, salt, or sugar by means of canning, pickling, smoking, curing, or fermentation.

- **Group 4:** Ultra-processed foods, which include sugar-sweetened beverages, sweet snacks, reconstituted meat products, pre-prepared frozen meals, canned soups, chicken nuggets, and ice cream. Processing in this category includes extraction and chemical modification. The end product contains very little food that is intact from group 1.[15]

In reading this, I'm sure that you're thinking group 4 sounds like something to be avoided at all costs. There are lots of negative connotations here. But let's dig deeper. Let's say you are a vegan and avoid animal products. Many products that would appeal to you (plant-based meat alternatives, plant-based milks) fall in the group 4 category. Does that make you unhealthy? Does that mean you should change your preference of avoiding animal products? Absolutely not. Or, to get even more drastic, let's say you or someone close to you is in the hospital and requires short-term tube feeding. Therapeutic fortified nutrition formula (for survival) falls into group 4. And for an everyday example, say you are a working parent, or better yet, just a busy adult. Life happens, and sometimes that means packaged or frozen meals that are quick and easy ways to nourish yourself. Yet all of those foods fit into group 4. Should you stop nourishing yourself? You get the idea.

There are many reasons why people choose the foods they do, whether they are packaged, canned, frozen, or fresh. Food choices are very individualized and depend on availability, preference, and dozens of other factors. There is no one size fits all. But the reality is that for many people, these foods are the only accessible means of nutrition, and they shouldn't be made to feel worse about what they eat. Because honestly, almost all food has nutrition. Although we are told over and over again to only ever eat fresh, organic produce, when you compare organic, fresh beans with a can of green beans, for example, you'll see very little difference in nutrients. The word *processed* causes mass panic, but according to the American Society for Nutrition (ASN), processed foods can provide sustenance to American diets because they contribute to food security—ensuring that sufficient food is available—and nutrition security—ensuring that food quality meets human nutrient needs.[16] The ASN also notes that food-processing techniques such as enrichment and fortification can add essential nutrients. So, what do these words mean? *Enriching* means adding the original nutrients back into processed foods, and *fortifying* means adding nutrients that would not have been there in the first place.[17] Doesn't really sound like a bad thing, does it? Processed foods don't need to be scary.

We choose the foods we eat for a variety of reasons—we don't just eat based on the nutrients that food provides. Affordability is one of those reasons, as many struggle to simply access food at all, let alone nutrient-dense options. Millions of Americans live in a food desert, which is a term used to describe societal inequities in access to food; it exists when at least a third of the population lives farther than one mile away from a supermarket for urban areas, or greater than ten miles for rural areas.[18] By this definition, 19 million Americans have limited access to a grocery store or supermarket. Every race in the country faces hunger, but systemic racial injustice means that African American, Latinx, and Native American communities are particularly prone to food insecurity and most frequently live in so-called food deserts— though perhaps the more accurate term is *food apartheid*. Coined by activist and farmer Karen Washington, the phrase *food apartheid* asks us to look at the root causes of inequity in our food system on the basis of race, class, and geography. Washington states, "Let's face it: healthy, fresh food is accessible in wealthy neighborhoods, while unhealthy food abounds in poor neighborhoods. 'Food apartheid' underscores that this is the result of decades of discriminatory planning and policy decisions."

Like affordability, accessibility is also a determining factor for our food choices. This can refer to the distance needed to travel for groceries but also how accessible a food is to make or open. Many packaged or canned foods are easier to manage for those with disabilities. Sixty-one million people in the United States live with a disability. About 13.7 percent have a mobility disability, meaning walking and/or climbing stairs can be difficult— which means it may be difficult to go shopping, a challenge that needs to be considered when discussing food access. Around 10.8 percent have a cognitive disability, which makes concentrating, remembering, and decision-making difficult, and those folks need something quick and easy to put together in order to get nourishment. And 6.8 percent have difficulty doing errands alone.[19] These tasks include but are not limited to shopping,

cooking, and food preparation, which includes opening packages. There are different types of packaging that make things easier to open and access. When it was originally marketed, Whole
Foods was trolled by some Internet users for selling peeled oranges in a container. But it had a purpose: folks who have trouble
with fine motor skills benefitted. Not to mention that many processed foods are often easier to swallow and digest for some folks.

Americans are particularly stigmatized for consuming ready-
made, packaged foods. There's the stereotype that America is so
unhealthy because of our food consumption. Let's rethink this—
bear with me here. Packaged foods provide convenience. Now,
why might Americans in particular need more convenience than
other countries? Let's look at our work-life balance here in the
States. Or maybe I should say lack thereof. We are very much a
hustle culture. Adults have packed schedules. Not everyone feels
like making a meal from scratch, wanting instead something that
saves time, and so they turn to packaged foods.

But let's unpack that more. Work-life balance refers to how
someone achieves balance in both their professional and their
personal life. What can happen if someone doesn't have a healthy
work-life balance? Burnout can occur, and that stress is one of the
most forgotten contributors that can impact our overall health.
What are some examples of this in action? Burning the midnight
oil even if you've left the office. Only 24 percent of employees
report never checking email after hours. So, 76 percent of people
are still checking in on work after they are off the clock.[20] So if
you're technically working after hours, do you have time to pre-
pare a meal from scratch? Chances are, no.

Further, 48 percent of Americans consider themselves workaholics.[21] America is one of just thirteen countries that don't guarantee paid time off for workers. How many times have you gone

on vacation and actually logged off? How many times were you fully present in where you were and what you were doing when not in the office?

And there are more statistics. Around 94 percent of workers in the professional service industry work over fifty hours a week.[22] Considering a regular workweek is about forty hours, that percentage is incredibly high. Let's throw in the idea that maybe you are responsible for young children. Again, I ask, are you thinking of making a meal from scratch? That box of Hamburger Helper is probably getting more and more appealing.

We tend to compare and contrast our lives and our health status here in the States to other countries, and the failing grade we give ourselves is real. But it doesn't just boil down to what we are and aren't eating. We are comparing ourselves to countries that celebrate food not just for its nutrients but for its social aspects. In many European countries, businesses close during lunch hours to give their employees proper time to prepare food and eat with their families. We could never imagine such a thing in the US. Further, many other countries have a health care system that guarantees care and supports mental health. Health is not solely what we are eating.

I'm going to emphasize that it's also more than okay to eat the foods you prefer. That's all. Believe it or not, preference is one of the factors in people choosing processed foods. We are fully allowed (not that we need permission) to eat foods that we like and enjoy. The end.

It's quite interesting how we casually refer to food as junk or garbage or use any other word that indicates a lower value. But a processed replacement shake can be a lifesaving way for someone to get nutrients and calories. That take-out dish, called a "cheat meal" and associated with the need to burn it off at the gym later on, is a celebratory food in someone's culture and has specific meaning. And that store-bought juice or cake was part of a celebration of love for some family. We don't just eat food for the nutrient content, and there are various ways to nourish the body. We also have to remember that nourishment of the soul is equally important.

CHAPTER FIVE

FOOD FREEDOM BEYOND "JUST EAT THE COOKIE"

You must always remember that the sociology, the history, the economics, the graphs, the charts, the regressions all land, with great violence, upon the body.
—Ta-Nehisi Coates[1]

I will never look down on someone for choosing to partake in a diet or restrictive way of eating. I'll repeat that I'm not, and I never will be, an anti-dieter. It's not my place to critique the food choices of others, because judging someone is the opposite of helping. What I am is antibiased and vehemently against a stigmatized society, especially when it comes to how we treat others based on food choices and bodies.

Now that we've got that straight, it's important to recognize some things. Changes in weight are a result of behavioral and/ or environmental changes. Loss isn't always positive, and gain isn't always negative. I hold space for those who want to contort their bodies, meaning I want folks to know that their concerns and thoughts are heard and recognized, because it is much easier to be accepted by society this way. I get it. It's easier to try to fit in than to constantly fight your way through. However, I personally will never suggest a restrictive diet—to anyone who asks—because I know they don't work and that the harm they cause almost always outweighs the good. When I work with clients, I also give information on the possible dangerous side effects of weight-loss medication and surgeries. But regardless of what folks are planning, I will never make someone feel as though they are making the wrong choice. I'm not living in their body.

People should feel empowered to know what's best for their bodies and for their lives. Yes, when making health decisions, we can seek professional opinions—and we should. But at the end of the day, every individual should make the choices that are best for their body. As a dietitian, I give people tools for their toolbox, and they can decide which are appropriate to use and when. Simply put, I believe in body autonomy. Body autonomy is the simple but radical concept that individuals have the right to control what does and does not happen to their bodies. United Nations Population Fund executive director Dr. Natalia Kanem describes it as "my body is for me; my body is my own. It's about power, and it's about agency. It's about choice, and it's about dignity."[2]

Many of us are over the endless cycle of dieting and the struggles that it brings. It's a weird feeling to chase this freedom, because many times we are met with "What about your health?" This is especially true for those in larger bodies. But choosing not to partake in dieting does not translate into not caring about your health. Choosing not to be overconsumed with the ingredients of your food does not translate into not caring about your health. It actually means the opposite: you are choosing to prioritize your mental health and you realize that the restriction and stress of dieting can be harmful.

In this same vein, weight is not a behavior. Correlation does not equal causation. There is no disease or illness that affects only larger bodies. Do we hear the opposite in the media? Yes, all the time. "*Obesity*" is frequently listed as a possible cause or factor of illness, but what often gets left out of the conversation is that weight stigma and biases from health professionals are also factors in determining outcomes. Having a larger body or being a higher weight is a simple correlation, not a causation, of a particular disease or illness.

• HEALTH AT EVERY SIZE •

So what constitutes actual health-promoting behaviors when we want to take our individual health into account? (The key word here is *individual* and realizing that we all have a unique blueprint.) As a dietitian, I personally align with Health at Every Size (HAES) principles and their weight- and size-inclusive approach to health. HAES was started in 2003 by the nonprofit organization Association for Size Diversity and Health (ASDAH). As of May 2023, it is described as a continually evolving movement that is an alternative to the weight-centered approach to treating clients and patients of all sizes. It promotes size acceptance and is on a mission to end weight discrimination and stigma and to lessen the cultural obsession with weight loss and thinness.[3] Not only does this movement promote size acceptance but it also acknowledges how the modern idea of health is weaponized and that we as a society place moral value on health. (Translation: the better health someone is in— or we assume they are in—the more value we place on them in society.) I want to also point out that according to ASDAH, their principles are constantly evolving and adjusting (as they should) with new information and leadership, which may change with time.

I believe that HAES is greatly misunderstood. I've seen countless tweets and posts on the topic that are sometimes grossly incorrect. For example, I gave a presentation a few years ago on the different ways we demonize food and shame those who eat in a certain way. My speaking points were part of a larger presentation about shaming, and I was presenting after a very prominent "obesity" research doctor. The irony, right? During one of our many meetings preparing for the event, the topic of HAES arose. I specifically remember the doctor talking us through the science of why and how we as humans crave and digest food. This is paraphrased, of course, but the gist of the conversation went something like this: "This is how we can see that obesity is a disease. This is what the HAES people don't understand." Obviously, my ears perked up, as an HAES-aligned dietitian. I also knew these words weren't directed at me, because this doctor had no idea of my alignment with the movement. There is absolutely nothing wrong with questioning things—I didn't start counseling with a weight-inclusive mindset. But I was open to learning and listening, and eventually my mind changed. This is my gripe with health professionals who consistently put it down. They are under the impression that HAES has a complete disregard for health, and that there is no concern with whatever illness or health-related issue someone has. That is not what HAES means. I'm effing tired of my colleagues having these close-minded thoughts and putting something down that they do not understand or care to understand.

There are ways to combat this mindset, though. The first step is addressing the language that is used. "*Obesity*" is a dehumanizing term to use, as many fat activists will continually explain.

As I mentioned in chapter 3, *obese* comes from the Latin *obesus*, which means "having eaten oneself fat." Many doctors today attempt to be more civil by saying "persons with obesity," which isn't any better. In providing the label of "obese," you are calling someone's body a disease. It's an inhumane way of addressing someone in a larger body or with a higher weight. Further, realize that, based on weight bias and stigma, some folks will never reach the level of health that society promotes. If you are constantly being discriminated against at the doctor's office and told to lose weight instead of your complaints being addressed, that is beyond a stigma—it's an act of violence against the individual. Not taking someone's ailments seriously can be fatal. Because this happens so often at medical offices, many folks in a larger body simply do not go to the doctor. Why would you intentionally go somewhere where violence is used against you? When you know that you will not be taken seriously? This is also why so many folks in a larger body do not love communal exercise environments. When society only upholds folks in thin bodies as the health standard (which many times is not true) it can make a pariah of anyone who doesn't fit that standard. Anyone larger is made fun of, mocked for daring to share the sacred space of fitness.

Another big misconception regarding HAES or other weight-inclusive practices is that it is only for folks in larger bodies. It most definitely is not, because it's called Health at *Every* Size; note the *every size* part. Everyone deserves equitable and unbiased care. As health professionals, we should be acknowledging our biases (we all have them) and providing information and services from an understanding of intersectionality that socioeconomic status, race, gender, sexual orientation, age, and other identities have an impact on our health. Remember the social determinants of health (SDOH), which we touched on earlier, will always impact our lived experiences. The biggest part of this movement comes down to respect, because so many—including health professionals, unfortunately—view a person's size as a pre-determining factor for how they are going to treat that individual.

In response to HAES, I see countless posts claiming that obesity is being glamorized. We need to keep in mind that not everyone is thin, and not everyone who loves and partakes in fitness and exercise is thin. Body diversity is real, and no matter what we do as a society to hide it, it's not going anywhere. I also can't help but notice that the level of outcry regarding emaciated bodies is not the same. The level of outcry for those who are damaging themselves with pills, starving, purging, and overexercising is near silent. These tactics that are actually unhealthy and dangerous and—depending on what social media page you stumble on—glamorized do not receive the same level of attention as the so-called obesity epidemic.

Letting go of diet culture does not mean letting go of your health. It means letting go of the idea that we all can achieve a certain aesthetic and saying goodbye to restricting and weight cycling; but more importantly, it's acknowledging that there is more to health than what we eat. Health is more than just genetics. It encompasses a system that is out of our control yet has deep roots in what makes us the individual humans we are.

• HEALTH INCLUSIVITY •

I personally like to subscribe to the eating for well-being principle of HAES. It's described as promoting flexibility and individualized eating based on hunger, satiety, nutritional needs, and pleasure rather than any externally regulated eating plan focused on weight control. What does this all look like in real life? How can we prioritize our health in a way that works for us and our needs? Because you need to eat. It's a basic human right and need. Unfortunately, there are quite a few hindrances for many in order to achieve that right. When I counsel, I always integrate the discussion of access to food in any talk of nutrition. This comes before speaking about illnesses and medical conditions, because it's pointless to discuss the foods someone should be eating without knowing if they can even access those foods. If someone is food insecure, they are more likely to be malnourished (which doesn't have a look and doesn't equate to emaciated), have chronic health conditions because they are not getting the nourishment they need, and have negative effects on their mental health, such as anxiety and depression.

Trauma can have a significant impact on our diet. It can lead to disordered eating habits, preoccupation with food, meal skipping, and/or lack of interest in food. The trauma can be long-term, and even if someone has overcome adverse experiences, the trauma can stay in their body and affect their present.[4]

There are so many intersectionalities with receiving non-biased health care, meaning there are multiple systems of inequality based on gender, race, ethnicity, sexual orientation, gender identity, disability, and class that are used as forms of discrimination. Therefore, there are multiple stigmas and biases that many others might face, and not being diagnosed and treated properly can happen to anyone with a marginalization. This happens frequently in a nutritionist's office, but I've also experienced it firsthand elsewhere. I'll never forget when I was in my midtwenties getting my annual checkup with a new OBGYN. Anyone with a vagina will know how awkward they are. I was sitting naked on the examination table with nothing but a thin sheet and my anxiety in the room. The doctor came in, and right away I felt an energy shift. Whether we can easily describe it or not, many of us can sense an energy exchange from others. This particular energy was not positive. This doctor was white, and we were probably around the same age, but I'll never forget the quick look up and down she gave me. To begin, I explained to her the issues I was having with my birth control medication. Without even looking at me, she said "Using protection helps." Umm, huh? There was no question, only an assumption. Mind you, I had already filled out the questionnaire and gone over this information with the nurse practitioner who asks about sexual history (which is standard). The implication threw me off. I sat there for a few seconds, flabbergasted, and just said, "Yes, I use it." Again, no eye contact. "How many partners do you have?" Yet another question that I had already answered with the nurse, and that information was in my patient profile, but the thing is, it wasn't really a question to get actual information. It was an accusatory question. Again I was stunned. "One." There was a pause when she finally looked at me and said, "Really?" And there it was. The confirmation that this wasn't an ordinary Q and A.

There will be some reading this thinking that I'm overreacting or that these are normal questions at the doctor's office. However, I can almost bet most of the marginalized folks reading this know this feeling and understand it quite well. These weren't normal questions. They were digs and microaggressions because of my race. This doctor was implying that a Black woman couldn't just have one partner (and there is absolutely nothing wrong with having more), and a Black woman was definitely not having safe sex. This directly correlates to how Black women are fetishized through misogynoir. The term *misogynoir* was first coined by writer and activist Moya Bailey, and it's defined as "the ways anti-Black and misogynistic representation shape broader ideas about Black women, particularly in visual culture and digital spaces."[5] There I was, being talked down to by a doctor because of learned stereotypes instead of my actual lived experience.

Now, I am a thin woman, but I still have the marginalized identity of being Black. There are multiple intersectionalities when we discuss biases and stigmas. I in no way know the feeling of weight stigma and the feeling of being in a doctor's office and being automatically dismissed due to weight. My understanding is from my lived experience of being dismissed because of my race. It was lazy, ignorant, and racist medical treatment. I have the same thing to say to health care practitioners who tell people to "just lose weight" for their ailments. It is lazy, ignorant, and fatphobic medical treatment.

Access to equitable and nonbiased health care is just one of the many determining factors that influence our health and overall well-being. There are so many factors that are out of our control, so it is mind-boggling when people in larger bodies are told to make better choices and that they don't care about their health. People do care—of course they do. It is extremely disheartening, however, to struggle to access nutritious food and clean water. It is also a struggle for those working multiple low-income jobs to feed their families. It's not noncompliance or not caring—it's systemic barriers that are often put in place.

• SOCIAL DETERMINANTS •
OF HEALTH AND ACES

Once I became a dietitian, I knew that I wanted to work in public health. I wanted to make a difference in the lives of those affected by systemic inequalities, because the environment plays a large role in our overall well-being and health—and because, for some people, there aren't better choices. Not acknowledging that is a form of healthism, and notions like "eat better," "just exercise," or "work harder" are all under this category.

Health professionals in particular should always ask ourselves why and what: Why are some people making the choices that they are making? What is preventing them from making certain decisions? Do they have access to a variety of foods, and if they do have access, are they able to purchase them? Let's bring in the SDOH we discussed in chapter 2; as a reminder, these are the conditions in the environments where people are born, live, learn, work, play, worship, and age that affect a wide range of health, functioning, and quality of life outcomes and risks.

Here's the wide variety of what some SDOH can look like in someone's life:

- Safe housing, transportation, and neighborhoods

- Racism, discrimination, and violence

- Education, job opportunities, and income

- Access to nutritious foods and physical activity opportunities

- Polluted air and water

- Language and literacy skills

Many of the aversions we face can begin when we are children. Adverse childhood experiences (ACEs) are potentially traumatic events that occur when we are young. ACEs and the associated toxic stress they create are strongly linked to nine of the ten leading causes of death in the United States. About 61 percent of adults reported they had experienced at least one type of ACE before age eighteen, and nearly one in six reported they had experienced four or more types of ACEs. The life expectancy of individuals with six or more ACEs is nineteen years shorter than that of individuals with none. ACEs can include abuse (physical, emotional, or sexual), neglect (physical or emotional), and/or household challenges (mental illness, incarceration, substance misuse, parental separation or divorce, or intimate partner violence).

ACEs are different from social determinants of health, but they are often interrelated, as SDOH factors might affect a child's health in certain situations. Insecure housing (SDOH) may leave families at risk for physical, emotional, or sexual abuse (ACEs). Increased carceral and law enforcement exposures contribute to adverse child mental health. ACEs and the associated SDOH can cause toxic stress, which can negatively affect brain development, immune systems, and stress response systems. Communities with lower incomes or higher crime rates may be overpoliced, leading them to be less desirable for investment and less likely to attract supermarkets with fresh foods. Communities with high neighborhood deprivation scores are more likely to have unclean air, water, and soil. Economic inequality often deprives these communities of the ability to build and transfer wealth and to weather health crises.[6]

Let's look further into economic and environmental inequalities by focusing on the accessibility of food options. Food is a human right, and we as a society often tell people to "eat better" and list different store options for people to shop at. Premium grocery chains that are focused on natural, organic, and specialty foods such as Whole Foods and Trader Joe's provide healthy shopping options, but also serve as markers of high-income, desirable areas; they contribute to increased property values and an image of security and stability. On the flip side, there are a large number of chain stores associated with poverty, such as dollar stores, that can indicate to investors and developers that a community is struggling or lacks a clientele that would make investment profitable.[7] Disproportionate access to food reveals the ways that society signals the value it places on the people in those communities.

While it might seem obvious that someone who experienced ACEs might be at risk in terms of health, many folks are still blamed for things that are out of their control. I'll never forget my experience during my dietetic internship. Note that in order to become a dietitian, one must complete an ACEND (Accreditation Council for Education in Nutrition and Dietetics) accredited supervised practice program (a dietetic internship) at a health care facility, community agency, or food-service corporation. The hospital I was assigned to was located in East Flatbush, Brooklyn, an area of New York where many inhabitants experience poor SDOH and are at risk for ACEs. While interning, I got to counsel patients one-on-one for the first time, and while I thought I knew what to expect before going in, nothing prepared me for some of my experiences. One day a weight consultation was requested for a patient who had type 2 diabetes. The patient was a Black woman whom I'll call Brittany (not her real name), who was about twenty-one years old and, according to the team, overweight. In Brittany's medical chart, one of the health professionals on the team had already described her as "difficult" and "noncompliant." Going into that consultation, I had built up some preconceived ideas of what to expect, including that this would probably be a waste of time. Brittany had been to the hospital before and was dismissive of recommendations. So why bother now? I walked into her room, and she was in the hospital bed listening to music on her earphones. I waved to her to signal I wanted to talk, and she immediately rolled her eyes and turned the music up. *Wow.* I had some choice words for her in my mind, but I stood my ground until she finally gave me her attention.

I asked her about her thoughts on the recommendations for food to help treat her type 2 diabetes. She shrugged. I was still very much a newbie, but I was determined to somehow get through to this woman. But because I was so new, I thought I knew what she needed and what would be best based on the advice from my textbooks, not from the lived experience in front of me. I asked what foods she liked and ate, figuring we could go from there. "I eat what I can at the shelter." I remember stopping and realizing the situation at hand. There was no note in her chart about being at a shelter, as she had used a family member's address on her intake forms, even though she didn't reside there. I asked if she had relayed any of this to the other staff; she had not. No one had cared to ask the whys and hows of her choices.

Brittany was homeless and had come from an abusive household, so she took what she was able to access. Many shelters do not take someone's personal needs into consideration. So no, she wasn't tailoring her dietary needs to her type 2 diabetes diagnosis. She didn't have safe housing, food access, or a stable income, and was going through significant trauma that was affecting her physicality. Difficult and noncompliant? How about tired of people judging her and giving her useless advice that wasn't applicable to her? Brittany did not need me to tell her how to eat and to lose weight. She needed a systemic solution. I spent the rest of the afternoon looking up Supplemental Nutrition Assistance Program (SNAP) benefits, food pantries, and soup kitchens. I also tried to think of agencies that could assist. By the time I went back up to her room the next day, she had been discharged. I remember the nurse telling me that she would probably be back in no time. I asked if anyone knew she was at a shelter and was met with, "Well, if she was so poor and not eating, how come she was so fat?" My head wanted to explode. This became a tipping point for my career in public health.

To provide a bit more context to that story, the demographic and socioeconomic factors in East Flatbush break down as follows: 84.2 percent of residents in East Flatbush are Black or African American (non-Hispanic).[8] Fifteen percent of adults in the neighborhood have diabetes, and 36 percent of adults have hypertension; stress and trauma from environmental factors play huge roles in these conditions.[9] And yes, racial trauma is a significant and important factor to acknowledge. In 2020, the American Medical Association named racism as a public health threat.[10] Dr. Camara Phyllis Jones, an American physician, epidemiologist, and antiracism activist who specializes in the effects of racism and social inequalities on health, defines racism as "a system of structuring opportunity and assigning value based on the social interpretation of how one looks (which is what we call 'race') that unfairly disadvantages some individuals and communities and saps the strength of the whole society through the waste of human resources."[11] So, what does this have to do with our individual health? It's a simple cause and effect.

Racism

Differential access to resources and differential living conditions

Chronic stress

Epigenetics (how behaviors and environment can cause changes that affect the way genes work[12]) and increased allostatic load (the cumulative burden of chronic stress and life events[13])

Health inequities
(cancers, heart disease, high blood pressure, etc.)

Traumatic experiences do not just occur externally; they also happen inside the brain and body. Stress causes the body to release cortisol, which increases heart rate and blood pressure, which can be useful for short-term threats. However, prolonged exposure to dangerously high levels of cortisol and chronic stress impacts the brain and can lead to increased medical comorbidities, such as diabetes types 1 and 2, coronary artery disease, and stroke.

We have not all been dealt the same hand in life. Social determinants of health come with adverse life experiences, and they have a significant impact on our health. Our health is not completely within our control. So no, telling someone to "just make better choices" when it comes to food is not helpful.

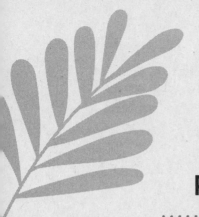

PART TWO

· ·

HOW TO MAKE NOURISHMENT WORK FOR YOU

CHAPTER SIX

INTUITIVE EATING

Release the idea of perfection, and know that every eating experience is an opportunity to get to know yourself better and discover what feels best in your body.
—Evelyn Tribole[1]

In 2018, I attended my first Food & Nutrition Conference & Expo (FNCE), an annual four-day event for food and nutrition professionals held by the Academy of Nutrition and Dietetics. It's basically the Coachella of the food industry—lots of mingling with peers, lots of learning from the educational presentations held throughout the day, and, of course, lots of free food samples available whenever you want. (I know that dietitians get a bad rap as the food police, but most of us really do love food! We get excited at the prospect of trying a variety of different foods. It's like five hundred times the samples that Costco hands out while you're shopping.) There are lots of educational talks about trending topics like gut health, malnutrition, and intuitive eating.

I was an eager newbie dietitian ready to immerse myself in the world of nutrition. That particular year, I went with two good friends who also happened to be newbie registered dietitians (RDs) and fellow career changers. We had no idea what to expect but were ready for the experience. Picture this: We're at the Pennsylvania Convention Center in Philadelphia in a sea of thousands of RDs and other nutrition and food professionals. It was overwhelming, exhilarating, and, honestly, intimidating. During the first couple of days, we even got lost trying to find presentation rooms and bathrooms, and when we finally found the room that we were looking for, there was usually a line to get in. While waiting on a line during day two, a friend stepped off quickly to use the bathroom, and when they came back, said, "Oh my god, Shana, you are so easy to spot in this crowd." I laughed because it was true. I stood out like a sore thumb. Mind you, this friend is Asian (and also knew me well enough to know that I would laugh at this), so they also understood the situation. Our profession is overwhelmingly white. That's not an exaggeration. As of this writing, I am part of the 3 percent of Black dietitians.[2] Some other numbers for dietitian ethnicity include 5 percent Asian and 6 percent Hispanic or Latinx. Think about what our society looks like in terms of demographics, and you can understand that 80 percent of dietitians being white is an alarmingly high number.

You're probably thinking, *I thought this chapter was talking about intuitive eating.* Trust me, this is going somewhere—because these statistics are important to keep in mind, and also this conference was my first introduction to the concept of intuitive eating. I had never heard of Evelyn Tribole or Elyse Resch, but, clearly, other attendees had. Their talk was held in a huge conference room that was packed. (My friends and I were a bit late and had to sit on the floor.)

The talk started with an overview of the Minnesota Starvation Study. Let's revisit this briefly, since we talked about it in chapter one. CliffsNotes: Thirty-six men volunteered in 1944 for a nearly yearlong experiment on the psychological and physiological effects of starvation conducted and monitored by Ancel Keys, PhD (this name might sound familiar to those interested in the Mediterranean diet), the physiologist in charge of the Minnesota lab. The lab's chief psychologist, Josef Brozek, PhD, was responsible for gathering the psychological data on the effects of starvation. The research protocol called for the men to lose 25 percent of their normal body weight. For the first three months the men were to eat a normal diet of 3,200 calories a day. (Yes, you read that correctly: a normal diet of 3,200 calories might seem shocking considering all the restrictive diets that are constantly being promoted. It sometimes seems as though anything more than 2,000 sends shock waves throughout society. Yet back in 1944, 3,200 was normal. I digress.) That would be followed by six months of semistarvation at about 1,570 calories a day. The semistarvation period was then followed by a rehabilitation period of three months of 2,000 to 3,200 calories a day, and then an eight-week unrestricted rehabilitation period during which there were no limits on caloric intake.[3]

Let's talk about the semistarvation phase. On the physical end, it resulted in gaunt appearances and significant decreases in strength, stamina, body temperature, heart rate, and sex drive. On the psychological end, hunger made the men obsessed with food. They dreamed and fantasized about it, read and talked about it, and savored the two meals a day they were given. There were also reports of fatigue, irritability, depression, and apathy. Does any of this sound familiar? Think about how you felt on your last diet.

This was one of the main points during the presentation that really hit me. The Minnesota study was one thing, but there are more than one hundred studies on the benefits of intuitive eating, not to mention that the concept itself has developed over the course of time. I had never really thought about how damaging restricting calories was—attending this presentation was eye-opening, as it started the change in how I viewed nutrition and its relationship to the body.

• INTUITIVE EATING IS NOT EATING •
WHATEVER YOU WANT

Without diet culture, intuitive eating would probably just be called eating. With all the rules and regulations that we are constantly given around food, it's not surprising that some of us need a framework to guide us back to a way of listening to our bodies. The stance at the heart of intuitive eating is that you are in control of your body and have the freedom to honor your hunger and food choices.

The definition of intuitive eating is as follows: "Intuitive Eating is a self-care eating framework, which integrates instinct, emotion, and rational thought and was created by two dietitians, Evelyn Tribole and Elyse Resch, in 1995. Intuitive Eating is a weight-inclusive, evidence-based model with a validated assessment scale and over 100 studies to date."[4] I think of this definition quite often because of the work I do with preschoolers. Part of my day job in public health is to visit preschools across New York City that fall into the low-income category and provide nutrition education. Nutrition education with three- and four-year-olds is quite the experience, and vastly different from an individual nutrition session with an adult. Preschoolers' nutrition education is more like providing fun facts, such as how a kiwi looks brown on the outside but is green inside. This seems nonsensical, but none of us woke up one day automatically knowing these things, and I will never not think how adorably amazed and wide-eyed children of that age get when they see a kiwi cut open in front of them. Aside from not being afraid to voice their opinions on foods and saying which ones they like and dislike (if you want to hear the truth, ask a preschooler), I am always amazed at the natural intuitiveness of their eating patterns. Part of the nutrition education at the public health program where I work encourages family-style dining in which everyone serves themselves. This is great for honing fine motor skills in still-developing children but also great for getting them to recognize their own hunger levels and how much they want and need.

One of the favorite food choices I provide are yogurt parfaits. I pass around a large bowl of yogurt, and each child spoons out their own helping. This can be nerve-wracking to watch at first. The portions they scoop out really vary. Sometimes they are small, and sometimes the kid has gotten so excited that they take too much. Even with this, the kids still know how much food they want. The kids who take too much always—and I mean always—stop eating when they're done. Even with foods they are clearly enjoying, they honor their fullness and stop. And almost always, any kid who takes too small a helping isn't afraid to ask for more. Children are notorious for being picky eaters, and while this is definitely true (and I know plenty of adults who are equally picky), children very much use their senses when they eat. They look at and feel the texture; they smell the food. Yes, there are some who have sensory sensitivities that come into play, but without realizing it, they are using something other than taste to determine their fondness for a food.

I share this because, unfortunately, what almost always happens is that this natural intuitiveness gets lost as we become

older. It can stem from our parents constantly pushing us to finish what's on our plates. If you were like me, you were part of the
clean-your-plate club growing up. Food costs money, and money
was not to be wasted—so even if you felt full, you ate everything
in sight. After all, there are starving kids in the world, so who are
we to throw away food? I'm sure this sounds familiar to many,
and it is one of the many reasons that those natural hunger cues
get distorted with time. It can also stem from the other end of
the spectrum, with parents pushing us to eat even though we
aren't hungry. You know that awkward moment when you're visiting family and you are full, but if you don't take what's being
offered, it's rude? That can also disrupt our hunger cues and mess
with our body's signals. It's not easy to balance what's good for
you and your body with social expectations, especially around
family. But we can try.

Full disclosure: I am not a certified intuitive eating counselor. I have the utmost respect for the concepts, which I
find beneficial, and I also model some of the same concepts
and non-diet approach in my own work. I own some of the
books, and I sometimes even recommend them to my clients
(depending on the situation). But while I think IE is great,
I also think there are holes. Privilege is very apparent in the
model (I appreciate that Tribole and Resch point this out themselves). IE is also overwhelmingly white, and I personally can't
fully identify with something that makes health and healthy
living seem accessible to everyone. Health is not accessible to
everyone because (here in the US, at least) we live in a society
that doesn't let everyone achieve the idea of health that we promote. Health is touted as a state that is completely illness- and
disease-free and is thought of as being in peak physical and
mental condition. This isn't possible for everyone, especially

for marginalized communities. Remember SDOH and racism being public health threats. Even as a thin, educated Black woman, I am not afforded the same level of health as my colleagues. If you scroll through #intuitiveeating on social media, you'll see endless numbers of white women promoting food freedom and how easy it is to just eat the cookie. Sometimes when I scroll through social media, I am reminded of my first FNCE conference. *Oh my god, Shana, you are so easy to spot in this crowd.* I relate to the content but at the same time I don't relate to it. It's very easy for my white, cisgender, able-bodied, and thin-bodied colleagues to smile and say just eat the cookie. There is privilege in saying that. Don't get me wrong—I fully believe in this statement, and I have used it myself. But it is frustrating to not see acknowledgment of healthism, white privilege, and social determinants of health.

And I know there will be some trolls reading this and thinking I am waging war on IE when in fact it's quite the opposite. I am acknowledging how helpful it is, while also acknowledging that it comes from a privileged mindset that I can't 100 percent align with.

• THE ORIGINS OF THE NON-DIET APPROACH •

Have you ever wondered about the origins of intuitive eating? When did the epiphany that restrictive dieting doesn't work occur? Because the term *intuitive eating* wasn't coined until 1995. There is indeed a history and an evolution of the non-diet approach to what it is today.

In 1973 Thelma Wayler, a registered dietitian, started the spa retreat Green Mountain at Fox Run, a weight-management program based not on dieting but on making smarter choices, eating well, moving one's body, and thinking positively. Wayler realized that diets and fads don't work and were not helpful with the "struggle with food and our bodies." In an interview with the *New York Times* in 1975 entitled "Don't Call It a Fat Camp," she noted, "We are educationally oriented all the way. What we are trying to do is change eating patterns for successful lifelong weight control."[5] Unlike the retreats that were being offered at the time, Green Mountain (which closed its doors around 2017) placed emphasis on nutrition education, a self-described intense program of physical activity, and an attempt at behavior modification through nutrition classes and group interactions that included activities such as free swimming, walking or jogging, golf, body conditioning, belly dancing, volleyball, exercising in the swimming pool, and more.

In 1978, Susie Orbach, a British psychotherapist, took it one step further and published a book called *Fat Is a Feminist Issue*. In her book, Orbach talks about how preoccupied we can become with eating, not eating, and avoiding fat. "When I sat down to write *Fat Is a Feminist Issue* forty years ago," she said, "I never dreamed, or feared, it would still be in print today. I naively hoped my book would change the world."[6] And it really did change the world. *Fat Is a Feminist Issue* explored how we can stop demonizing food and find ways to accept ourselves for who and how we are. "The preoccupation with the body and the fact that there are industries that make so much money out of women's discontent, and now men's; the diet industry, the fitness industry, the cosmetic industry, these are all huge businesses. They sell an aspirational position where we have to appear in a certain way," Orbach said in a 2015 interview with the *Irish Times*.[7] Personally, I find it sort of wild to see how history repeats itself.

Many of the same issues and events that we have gone through as a society haven't changed in a really meaningful way. We are still talking about dieting and contorting the body. We are still within the mindset that fat is bad and thin is good and that there is a morality attached to it.

Despite the social upheaval of the 1970s, there was still media messaging and societal pressure to adhere to an ideal body—the thin body type. The incidence of severe anorexia nervosa requiring hospital admission rose significantly during the 1960s and '70s.[8] In the same *New York Times* article about Thelma Wayler, one of the participants at the retreat stated that she thought some women got fat because they tended to refuse the role of what they were supposed to be, "a sex object . . . to reduce the pressures put on thin, attractive women." Mind you, this movement was happening at the same time that the feminist movement was in full swing, and women were wanting more than traditional gender roles.

In 1982, Geneen Roth's first book, *Feeding the Hungry Heart*, was described as "how Geneen Roth remembers her time as an emotional overeater and self-starver."[9] Roth's books regarding food and eating often link compulsive eating and perpetual dieting with deeply personal and spiritual issues that go beyond food, weight, and body image. For more than thirty years, she has been speaking, teaching groundbreaking workshops, and offering retreats.

Needless to say, it has been quite a journey to what we now know as intuitive eating and the series of books that started in 1995. IE has gained intense popularity (which makes it all the more amusing how out of the loop I was at FNCE), so much so that it has even been co-opted by the weight-loss sector. "Intuitively lose weight!" Nope, not a thing, at least if you're abiding by the official IE guidelines and principles. Let's run through some brief notes on IE and its ten principles, from the fourth edition of *Intuitive Eating*, which I have taken and recapped with some of my own approaches.[10] I will shamelessly add that I also own this book. See, I'm not a hater.

Principle 1: Reject the Diet Mentality

The first, and probably the most challenging, principle is to reject the diet mentality. The diet industry is an industry, after all, and its end goal is always making money. This realization can be extra difficult because diet culture is sneaky and infiltrates every part of our lives. It's not just the Weight Watchers ads that we see. It's also in the television shows that promote the same narrative or social media that constantly pushes a certain aesthetic. Plus, many of these fixtures of diet culture are now rebranded as lifestyle changes and/or aspects of a wellness plan. Not to mention that the intuitive eating language has been co-opted and used to promote weight loss, which—news flash—is the antithesis of intuitive eating. And if the theme of any plan or advice being given is rooted in restriction, then it's not intuitive eating, it's a diet.

The first principle is described as "Throw out the diet books and magazine articles that offer you false hope of losing weight quickly, easily, and permanently. Get angry at diet culture that promotes weight loss and the lies that have led you to feel as if you are a failure every time a new diet stopped working and you gained back all the weight."

This is actually quite scary for some people, because rejecting the mentality and really preparing yourself to be free of diets means that you have to begin trusting yourself when you have been told consistently that you cannot trust yourself or your body. When undertaking this step, I always recommend doing a social media detox. This means unfollowing or muting posts that highlight weight loss or restrictive eating in any capacity. We aren't always attuned to the constant messaging we are receiving. It's obvious when it's a direct ad on our television but we are sometimes desensitized to the influencers promoting this rhetoric. Be mindful.

Principle 2: Honor Your Hunger

How many times have we all felt that pang in our stomach signaling that we feel hungry? But instead of stopping to eat we think there's no way we can be hungry because we ate recently. Or maybe in our minds it's too early to eat because we feel as though we just ate breakfast or lunch. Sometimes we honestly don't feel our hunger because of stress, medications, or past traumas that have altered our internal signals. Denying our body food when food is necessary for our survival is not honoring our hunger. Further, we should not base our hunger or food intake on that of others— that's an easy way to deny our individual body cues.

We also should acknowledge that there are different types of hunger. There is the physical hunger that we feel when we receive the signals that our bodies give us. Mind you, these signals aren't always stomach growls. They can come in the form of tiredness, lack of concentration, irritability (hangriness), and much more. Our bodies are constantly talking to us and giving us signals.

There's also taste hunger, which can be described as simply wanting food because it sounds good. This could happen at a friend's birthday celebration that ends with cake, a holiday potluck at work, or maybe when your mom wants you to try the zucchini bread that she spent the morning baking (yes, this is

100 percent my mom). We don't feel hunger and definitely feel fullness, but we still have the desire to taste. This is all normal and not wrong.

Practical hunger is for those days when we know our schedule is going to be wonky—back-to-back meetings, on-the-go appointments. Whatever is going on, you know that your day is going to be hectic, and you might have to spend more time planning for your meals, or you might not be able to just wait to eat when you're hungry. You might have to just eat something because you realize that your next opportunities will be few and far between.

And then there's emotional hunger, which we relate to eating our feelings or seeking comfort food. When we have negative thoughts around food being comforting, we still tell ourselves that food should be eaten for its nutritional value only. Food represents many aspects outside of nutrients, and there is a sense of familiarity and comfort that comes with certain foods. This doesn't make the food wrong. It's okay to nourish your soul.

Principle 3: Make Peace with Food

You know that feeling when you are about to start yet another diet and you are faced with the harsh reality of all the foods on the do-not-eat list, and so you do what any normal human does and panic eat (binge) the forbidden foods because you won't have access to them soon? This is a very real phenomenon called the Last Supper effect. It is a familiar feeling for many because we tend to place foods in a hierarchy. Diet culture instills in us that there are good foods and bad foods.

Reminder: food has no moral value. Therefore, the concept of food neutrality—which I interpret as viewing food as neither superior nor inferior, because all foods provide some form of benefit—is incredibly important because of our tendency to equate our actions with our moral worth. That's often why we use phrases such as "I'm being so bad" when we want to order dessert. And follow it up with "I promised myself I would be good" when we order a salad out of penance for having said dessert the night before. It sounds innocent, but how we talk to ourselves in relation to food is so important to the concept of IE. You need to have a neutral view toward food and realize that no, cookies (and all sweets/desserts, for that matter) are not bad. We can still eat cookies and be good.

I can hear it: *But if I allow myself to have cookies in the house, I will eat them all at once.* One of the hardest realizations is that the very same foods we don't allow ourselves freely are the ones we feel like we have less control over. This means not deeming certain foods to be special foods or treats. Practicing this can be scary, because at first it can feel like you are out of control, constantly wanting the foods that had been off-limits. But eating that food does not make you bad. What we eat doesn't determine our worth as humans.

Principle 4: Challenge the Food Police

We are our own worst critics. The pressure we put on ourselves—to abide by rules, to be perfect when it comes to eating—can hinder us in achieving food neutrality. Plus, sometimes we don't even realize that we have rules. Here's a few I've heard: can't eat past 7:00 p.m.; no more than two carbs at a meal; no starchy vegetables. These are arbitrary rules that we often give only to ourselves, and when we break said rules, we keep tabs and hold ourselves accountable.

This accountability takes the form of guilt and stress, which can cause havoc in our bodies in the form of pain, bloating, nausea, and other stomach discomforts. In other words, these things are not helpful. Even though the word *dieting* is no longer in vogue, we still follow arbitrary rules and regulations under the umbrella of *wellness*. We often talk ourselves out of eating and nourishment in favor of policing ourselves.

There is no one way of eating that works for everyone. Following a list of dos and don'ts that others abide by is not only unnecessary but also unhelpful. It causes us to go against our unique biological signs and signals. Recognizing that nothing is black and white and there is a ton of gray can be helpful. Instead of feeling discouraged because you can't seem to follow the no-eating-past-7:00-p.m. rule, maybe realize that your work schedule requires you to work until 6:00 p.m., after which you go for a run to relax. This might mean eating after 7:00 p.m., which isn't wrong for you as an individual. In fact, it may be what your body needs.

Principle 5: Discover the Satisfaction Factor

We have taste buds for a reason. And thanks to diet culture, we forget how pleasurable food can and should be. We're conditioned to think that when food is delicious, it has to be bad. If we enjoy something too much, it has to be wrong.

Try to use your senses when eating. What does something taste like? Notice whether something is sweet, salty, sour, or bitter. Is the taste actually pleasurable to you, or are you consuming out of habit? What is the texture like? Is it crunchy, chewy, or smooth? Many times, a food can be unappealing to us because of the texture. What do you smell? Think about the last time you walked past a bakery and smelled the aroma of fresh bread. Is it pleasant? Are there foods that are off-putting in smell? What about the temperature? Hot soup might be undesirable on a one-hundred-degree day. Ice cream might be undesirable when it's snowing.

Really think about why you like certain foods. Is it actually satisfying you when you use your senses? I often think about a brand of yogurt that I used to buy during my dieting years. I ate it out of habit and never concentrated on whether I actually enjoyed it. Even after I told myself I was done with diets, I still ate it because it was familiar. It was only after I embraced this principle and really used my senses that I discovered I did not like the taste at all. After that, I started eating a yogurt brand that was actually satisfying to me.

Principle 6: Feel Your Fullness

We have all eaten past fullness at some point in our lives. There are numerous reasons behind this, none of which make us inferior humans. So much of how we ate as children can be reflected in how we eat as adults. Factors include food insecurity, poverty, other adverse childhood experiences, or being part of a clean-plate household.

It can often be hard to feel our fullness. One way to help is to be fully present. It's easier said than done. It was personally one of the hardest things for me to learn, and I'm still not perfect at it. And, of course, there is no such thing as perfect eating. Being present means continually checking in with yourself on your satiety during meals. Take a moment and ask yourself, are you still hungry? What is your hunger level now? If we are distracted when eating, we can mindlessly inhale our food. Eating without distractions can feel strange at first because we are used to juggling tasks and thoughts, but if you find yourself having difficulty feeling your fullness, this might be worth a try. Check in and really gauge your hunger throughout the meal. There is no wrong answer here. Some days you are going to realize that you need more food. Some days you might realize that you need less.

Principle 7: Cope with Your Emotions without Using Food

With all this talk about honoring our hunger, we also need to address emotional eating. Food is more than a source of nutrients; it can also be used to quell whatever feelings we're having. It's instant gratification that we use for a dopamine hit because we want a distraction.

There have been many times while writing this book when I wanted to procrastinate instead of actually sitting down and getting all these thoughts out. I was stressed, nervous, and anxious about writing. Making snacks was a great distraction from what I really needed to be doing. I used food more than once to quell my uneasy thoughts. Why am I telling you this? Because perfection doesn't exist. It's important to recognize these scenarios and think about other steps to take. Other emotions can include being excited, angry, and bored. These are all perfectly valid emotions, and there is nothing wrong with having them. However, we can try to find coping mechanisms other than food to address them.

Writing in a journal, calling a friend, and going to therapy are great ways to get out our emotions if we are feeling stressed about a certain situation. Crossword puzzles, reading a book, and DIY crafts are some great ideas for when we're feeling bored. Having a healthy relationship with food entails realizing that food can be pleasurable. We should eat foods we enjoy, but there is a difference between truly loving and savoring a dish or a food and using it to cope with unresolved feelings where we aren't even tasting or truly enjoying it.

Principle 8: Respect Your Body

"You don't have to like every part of your body to respect it." We all have our bad days, and this is normal. But what we can do is respect our bodies by not attempting to contort ourselves for a certain aesthetic. We tend to put ourselves on the back burner when it comes to care. We are used to making sure that our loved ones are taken care of, fed, and nourished, but often don't extend that care to ourselves. Even pets are better maintained than we are ourselves, because we would never deny them food, movement, and treats. How often do we think to do that to ourselves?

This is easier said than done, especially for those who are in a larger body. Focusing on improving someone's actual health rather than focusing on weight is actually health promoting. We already covered HAES in chapter three, so as a recap, recall that using a weight-centric approach only contributes to food and body preoccupation, weight cycling, a decrease in self-esteem, and eating disorders. Respecting your body also includes eating for well-being, which incorporates an individualized approach based on hunger, nutritional needs, pleasure, and satiety. Physical activity means finding ways to move that you truly enjoy. These are ways we can respect ourselves, because no matter what, our bodies deserve nourishment.

Principle 9: Movement—Feel the Difference

I can't tell you how many fitness classes I have taken that I wasn't enthusiastic about. I simply felt guilty not going or was peer pressured into attending. And as a surprise to no one, I slowly began to skip sessions and then stopped going altogether. I used to think there was something wrong with me personally for not having the willpower to stick it out. I mean, everyone else liked being yelled at by the screaming instructor, so obviously the issue was me. I was still equating movement with burning calories and not actually with its other health-promoting benefits. I was separating exercise and joy as though they were different categories.

There are many benefits to movement that aren't about weight reduction. These include an increase in bone strength, a decrease in blood pressure and stress, an increase in heart and lung strength, improved memory, and much more. The best movement isn't the one that's the hardest, it's the one that is the most enjoyable and that you can do joyfully. As a New Yorker, walking is my jam. I am thankful to live in a walkable city, and I take advantage of it by walking everywhere I can. It helps clear my head, it's sometimes quicker than public transportation, and it helps me physically. Is it the most challenging or difficult activity? No, absolutely not, but I find that it is a favorite of mine. Additionally, since I've recovered from my disordered eating days, I have reevaluated my love of dance and found actual joy in it again. Bottom line: it doesn't matter how small, every activity counts and can be beneficial.

Principle 10: Honor Your Health with Gentle Nutrition

As we've noted, intuitive eating is not eating whatever you want and disregarding health. Instead, it means honoring your body by nourishing it with nutrients and also acknowledging preferences and taste buds. When we start adopting a food-neutral approach, a salad isn't penance for eating a burger the night before. Plain steamed vegetables don't have to be the only vegetable option that offers nutrition. When we truly get in touch with our bodies, we can listen and learn what they need.

I love salads. I love the crunchiness of the greens and the different flavors of the other produce I put in, including fruits, vegetables, and grains. I like the way my body feels when I'm eating it. But I'm never going to say that it's superior to ice cream, because when I want something creamy and sweet, salad ain't cutting it. I can listen to what my body wants and needs. There will always be other factors that can override our natural intuitiveness like stress, trauma, and medications, but we can start to really honor our bodies by learning how to nourish individually.

• INTUITIVE EATING DOES NOT HAVE • TO BE THE END

IE is a great framework, especially if you are beginning your non-diet approach. However, in my work, I think that it is important to add to these principles and realize they may not resonate with everyone. Not everything works for everyone. It's 100 percent okay if something is not fully aligning with you.

This is coming from someone who was mesmerized when I first learned about IE and began to rethink my own approach.

I considered becoming a certified IE counselor because I was committed to the framework. But when I began to counsel clients on my own, I realized that IE was not as perfect as I thought. I had a client once who was having issues with the framework because she was getting frustrated about following the principles. As someone who had just gone through years of extreme dieting, it was difficult for her to not compare following the IE principles to following the rules of a diet. She had a history of dieting and extreme poverty. She had anxiety and attention deficit hyperactivity disorder (ADHD). For her, this framework was not complementary, and that was okay. So we threw out the principles and started from scratch. And this was not a one-off case—I've had lots of clients who need to work outside of IE.

As I mentioned before, IE also has a very white, cisgender, nondisabled, and neurotypical dominant mindset. I follow the same non-diet approach, but there is something unnerving about white women posting "Just eat the cookie!" and not acknowledging that many of us cannot intuitively eat our way out of the systemic racism that affects our health. Those who are transgender cannot intuitively eat their way out of the fear of being violently assaulted. I can't help but get aggravated at the thought of nearly every white colleague remaining politically neutral out of fear of losing followers when health is political. How can I fully align with this when being a Black woman is a literal risk factor due to systemic barriers? Allyship and support is more than a black square on Instagram (circa June 2020) or a post with some Black creators on Juneteenth or Black History Month. It means acknowledging privilege and actively working on change.

This is at the heart of the reason why I decided not to become IE certified. No one way of eating works for everyone, and it is our job as dietitians to work with folks on an individual level. There is no such thing as perfect. What I will do in the following chapters is go through my way of thinking and my recommendations regarding food. And guess what? This is not going to work for everyone. That's more than okay. This is just to show you some examples.

CHAPTER SEVEN

FIND YOUR OWN PATH

We are not all in the same boat. We are all in the same storm.
Some of us are on superyachts. Some have just the one oar.
—Damian Barr[1]

Despite what diet culture tells us, we should eat for a variety of reasons: our health needs, preferences, hunger, and pleasure. Yes, pleasure—heaven forbid we enjoy the food we are eating! There are many activities—like sex or various forms of movement—that we partake in for pleasure and not just their socially accepted health benefits. Eating should be one of those!

In order to get to this happy place of eating for pleasure and joy, we also need to accept and respect our predetermined genetics and other external factors. I might sound fantastical, I know. But imagine eating what you want to, in a way that is individualized for your needs. And I don't just mean needs in terms of calories or nutrients; I mean eating foods that make you feel good, emotionally and physically.

Sounds sort of radical, doesn't it? We aren't supposed to eat what we want—we're supposed to follow diet rules because we have been taught not to trust our own bodies and desires. There are more than eight billion people on this planet, with radically different needs and body types, and yet we still somehow believe there is one magical way of eating that will work for everyone, that there is some perfect regimen we will all be able to stick to and that will get us all looking pretty much the same. But imagine if we didn't have a thin ideal for what a body should look like. Imagine if we universally accepted the concept of body diversity. Imagine if we all ate for our own individualized well-being.

In the previous chapter, we talked about intuitive eating, an approach that emphasizes food freedom. But given how immersed we are in the rules of diet culture, even the concept of intuitive eating can feel like yet another diet for some. After all, those principles can feel a lot like rules, particularly if you're coming from years of restrictive dieting. I'm not a certified Intuitive Eating counselor but I do understand the principles, and I find that it is helpful for some clients as a starting-off point to undo the damage of years of restriction. In a way, intuitive eating principles serve as reminders of how we should look at food and eating as a whole.

Within this, there is always talk of food freedom and getting to a place of feeling unrestricted in terms of how and what to eat. When you go on social media there are countless posts of "just eat the doughnut" or "don't be afraid of whole milk in your coffee" under the #foodfreedom tag. Let me be clear: I agree with these statements wholeheartedly; however, they can be frustrating when you are trying to reclaim your instincts surrounding food because that's neither something that magically happens overnight nor is it second nature. Food freedom can be a difficult concept to grasp, and even more difficult to embody in our everyday lives. We've discussed how stress and trauma can throw off hunger cues. ACEs like poverty can also play a role in how we view and experience food. How can someone find food freedom or eat intuitively when they don't have access to food? How can someone access their intuition if their childhood was spent not receiving enough food or feeling guilt around food? Further, if you have allergies or intolerances, food freedom can feel like an impossible goal. I regularly post about the concept of food freedom (of course making sure to include the intersectionality of SDOH and ACEs) on social media and am always hit with comments like "What about my allergies?" or "What about my [insert medical condition]?" I have multiple food allergies, so I know the feeling of having to go over every detail of the ingredient list on packages, not to mention having to double-check menu items when dining out. Trust me when I say this: it does not feel like food freedom. Even so, I believe that food freedom is often unfairly seen as an all-or-nothing choice.

Food freedom doesn't mean everybody gets to eat whatever they want with no consequences. If you decided to eat nothing but pints of ice cream all day, how would that make you feel? I mean, ice cream is delicious, yes, but how would our bodies actually feel at the end of the day if that's what we decided to subsist on? What would our energy levels be? If you know that a certain amount of dairy won't be kind to your stomach, maybe that's something to consider. Would ice cream be sustainable and accessible throughout the day if you commute to work? Probably not. I use the example of ice cream, which might sound ridiculous, but you can run through any scenario that applies to you personally. Think about what your day-to-day life looks like. The media will tell you to avoid packaged foods, but are those foods what help you to nourish yourself in the morning? If you need a granola bar or portable yogurt to get you out of the house in the morning, that's okay. The influencer walking through a grocery store tells you that he doesn't snack all day so you shouldn't either, but you're the one working a twelve-hour shift in a hospital. If you are preparing for your day with portable snacks and with packaged meals, that is actually eating intuitively.

Food freedom means eating in a way that works for you, which includes taking into account your personal preferences—likes and dislikes—as well as your cultural foods, lifestyle factors, and economic status. That means not following anyone's rules, or even setting your own rules. It means figuring out what works best for you and what doesn't. It means not having to feel like a failure if you get off track. It means allowing yourself to eat unconditionally and not needing to log anything into an app or device or waiting until a certain time to eat.

If you're used to following rules around eating, this can be pretty difficult. I mean, haven't we all been there? Like when it's 10:15 a.m. and you're hungry but it's too early for lunch (who made up this time rule?), and you feel like you shouldn't be hungry in the first place since you just ate breakfast at 8:30. So you wait to eat and ignore your growling stomach because those are the rules. Let's step back and look at what's really going on here. You're ignoring your body's hunger cues, but why? The first reason is time—you feel like you have to wait until a certain time to eat, because we are taught from a young age that lunch starts around noon. This is an external cue that is totally arbitrary but that we feel obliged to follow. Also, you may feel a certain shame that you already feel hungry again. But if your breakfast was a tiny container of yogurt and coffee, then yes, I imagine your stomach is going to be rumbling. Even if it was an egg and spinach wrap, your hunger is still real, because your energy needs (calorie needs) vary from day to day. You should feel free to eat to satisfy it without guilt or shame.

• HOW TO NOURISH YOURSELF •

Let's talk about how to nourish yourself. The key word here is *yourself*; you don't need to follow what a celebrity is doing or your spin instructor suggests. You are different and have different needs. The below are some food-for-thought affirmations to help get you started on this journey.

Food for Thought 1: The only foods to avoid are those that you're allergic to, must avoid for medical reasons, or don't like.

Do you ever notice that when you ask someone about the fad diet they're doing and inquire why they are avoiding certain foods, they usually don't have a clear answer? "You know . . . inflammation." "To clear up the toxins." "I just feel better." Shout out to the MVPs who will actually say, "I don't know, I read that Blake Lively [or some other random celeb] cuts out soy, so I'm trying it." There is nothing wrong with being curious about the lifestyle choices of others, especially a favorite celebrity or influencer. I get it; I do. We like these people, and we may look up to them. But what we often forget is that our bodies are completely different from theirs. Well, I think we do know this on some level, but it's easy to hold some underlying hope that our bodies will transform to mimic theirs, especially if we share some of their characteristics. Let's say you are the same height, weight, and body type as Gabrielle Union. Even then, you are not going to have the same exact results from eating like she does. Our bodies all process foods differently. And let's not forget that these celebrities we aspire to look like are on a completely different financial level than almost everyone else, and maintaining their bodies is a large part of their jobs. They have an enormous amount of time and resources to put toward their appearance, which is just not realistic for most of us. (Not that this makes it any more okay; the Hollywood pressure to be thin still stems from fatphobic culture.)

Most fad diets use buzzwords like inflammation, toxins, gut health, imbalance, and more. The words tend to sound pretty scary (that's the point), and they can be a real issue for some people. But do they all apply to you? Not necessarily. There are so many factors that impact our health, and any messaging that implies that cutting out one or two specific foods will cure everything is extremely misleading and potentially harmful. Body size, genetics, chronic illness, chronic stress, level of income, hormones, medications, and trauma all impact how we eat and how our bodies process food. So the next time you decide to cut out a certain food or food group because you heard it's the latest diet trick, stop and ask yourself why you're really doing it. Are you allergic? Do you have a medical reason not to eat that food? Is it a food you don't like? If the answer to all of these questions is no, stop to reconsider. Cutting out gluten or soy might solve some issues for you . . . but it might not. Try to look at the whole picture rather than avoiding a food you enjoy just because someone told you it can cause inflammation.

Food for Thought 2: Food is food.

Food isn't good, bad, toxic, sinful, clean, guilt-free, indulgent, or any other fun adjective that the wellness industry likes to come up with. Food has no moral value. Food is food, meaning it provides energy to you in the form of calories. We have been taught to fear calories, and that we should eat as few as possible. But here's the thing: calories are units of energy. That's actually their definition. We as functional human beings need energy in order to get through the day, let alone thrive. Calories are essential to life. If we eat 400 calories of food, that is 400 units of energy that our body can use. Now, here's the part that folks might forget: our bodies don't just need calories for movement and exercise. Our bodies need them for everyday living. We all have a basal metabolic rate (BMR), which is the baseline number of calories we need just to function. And no, the number isn't zero. Our bodies need about 1,300 calories alone just for our organs to function. Our brain needs 240–320 calories. Our liver, 200 calories. Our heart, 440 calories. And our kidneys, 420 calories.[2] That's 1,300 calories total, more than what some diets allow for a daily limit.

That's why the idea of 1,200 calorie diets (1,200 calories is what toddlers need, by the way) is so infuriating. Consuming less than your BMR is dangerous, and it will cause your body to go into survival mode.[3] Ever wonder why you were so cranky and irritable on your last low-calorie diet? This is why. You were starving. Literally.

We need calories to survive, calories we get from food—any food. There are nourishing foods that will provide you with different nutrients, but everything you eat provides something for your body. It's okay if that something is comfort or pleasure. We have taste buds, after all, and it's normal for us to want to hit every part of our palate.

Dividing foods into the categories of good and bad only perpetuates the idea that you are a good person if you eat something you are told is healthy and that you are a bad person if you eat something you are told is unhealthy. This is the last thing you need. Guilt is not a side dish or an ingredient that belongs anywhere near food. In order to get to a healthy relationship with food, it's important to try to let go of these misleading labels and to remind yourself that food is food. Full stop.

Food for Thought 3: Think of eating in terms of addition rather than subtraction.

You don't have to restrict the foods you enjoy. In fact, I highly recommend that you don't do this, because it will likely make you crave those foods even more. For example, one of my first clients claimed that she ate "like a twelve-year-old." She was nervous about seeing me, assuming a dietitian would immediately tell her to forgo her favorite foods. Even though she knew my stance as an anti-diet dietitian, this was still her biggest fear. She explained that she loved ramen noodles. And not the fancy restaurant or DIY kind but the ninety-nine-cent kind that college kids stock up on because they're "cheap" and quick. (I will always put "cheap" in quotations because everyone's finances are different, and this might not be cheap for some.) I could see her cringing as she told me this, bracing herself for some kind of reprimand for liking something so obviously unhealthy. She was completely shocked when I said, "Okay, great, let's keep that in."

Why was this my response? Well, she shared that store-bought ramen noodles were something that she loved. She had a busy work schedule, and ramen was easy. Why would I take that away from her? Let's think back to the last Food for Thought. Was this something she didn't like to eat? Nope. Was this something that she was allergic to? Obviously not. Was this something that she should have restricted for medical reasons? No. And for all of you thinking about diabetes (which someone will always bring up when talking about carbs) or any other condition for which carbs are the enemy, you still don't have to completely restrict them.

Many clients I see who are diagnosed with diabetes are told by their doctors to stop eating carbohydrates altogether, and in my opinion, that's just lazy counseling. For one, doctors are not nutrition experts. Second, eating with diabetes involves planning and timing with meals, not restricting a whole food group.

Ramen noodles are comforting and delicious, as food should be. But as a dietitian, I also want some nourishment in there in the form of protein, fiber, and healthy fats. That's where math comes in. Instead of cutting out the ramen, I told her to try thinking of nourishing foods to add to her noodles. Still feeling guilty about eating like a twelve-year-old, she was reluctant to say she preferred broccoli, because apparently that's the vegetable of choice for kids. Who knew? But you know what broccoli is full of? Fiber; vitamins K, C, B, and A; calcium; protein; potassium; and antioxidants. I listed all these great benefits and her face lit up. Adding a food like broccoli is what I refer to as bulking up a meal. And, mind you, it doesn't have to be fresh, organic anything—stock up on frozen or canned vegetables and you can quickly and easily bulk up your meals without spending lots of money.

This method can work with any meal or snack. You can add fruit to your breakfast in cereal, on top of toast, or on the side. Chopped vegetables can be added to eggs. Lettuce, tomatoes, cucumbers, apple slices, pear slices, and onions can all be added to sandwiches. Vegetables can also be added to stir-fries, pasta dishes, and casseroles. You feel insecure about messing around with a recipe by adding things in? Try just having something on the side—and yes, it can be prepackaged, canned, or frozen. Ready-made salads are quick and easy, and there's nothing wrong with them. And remember, just because a food is nourishing doesn't mean it has to be boring or bland. I often think sometimes we just aren't told how to make something tasty. That's why so many adults suddenly love a variety of different foods, such as different vegetables, later in life. We finally adulted and learned how to make them!

Food for Thought 4: The way you eat isn't a personality trait.

Have you ever met someone at a party or other event and they start telling you about how they've started keto and are intertwining it with intermittent fasting? When people embark on fad diets, it seems to become one of their personality traits. This makes sense, as fad diets are built on rules that leave no room for error. When we are engaged in such a culture, we want to talk about it in order to feel some sort of validation.

Keto. Weight Watchers. Noom. Paleo. Whole30. South Beach. Atkins. Intermittent fasting. These are all names that people attach their identities to. But how you eat doesn't have to have a fancy name in order to be valid—and it's also no one else's business. Not to mention that over the years, our needs change. This is normal, and part of listening to our own bodies and not adhering to guidelines or fads just because everyone else is.

Maybe you realize that if you go to bed at 9:30 p.m., you need to stop eating at 8:00 p.m. for your body to respond best. Notice how I specifically wrote "your body"? Good. You don't need to label it intermittent fasting and then try to only eat between 12:00 p.m. and 8:00 p.m. (or whatever time frame). Eating only within certain hours because that's what you've been told to do is another way of adhering to a diet—which makes it unnecessarily restrictive. Maybe you realize that sweet potatoes upset your stomach for some reason and decide not to eat them. Totally valid, because who wants to walk around with a stomachache? But does this mean you need to cut out all starches and follow something restrictive like keto? No. Picking a label and going extreme is just not necessary.

I know that going through the process of figuring out what works best for your body and building trust with yourself doesn't sound as sexy as doing the next fad diet. But my point is that we don't need to constantly label the way we eat. It doesn't have to be a personality trait. When in doubt, go back to Food for Thought 1.

Food for Thought 5: Stop hating on packaged foods.

I'm asking nicely here, with a really big smile on my face. Seriously, though, why so much packaged food hate? I know that part of it is because we live in an elitist society. Are there foods that are processed? Yes, definitely. In fact, just about everything we eat is. Are all processed foods less nourishing? No. That bag of raw spinach is processed. That package of organic cacao is also processed. As is that box of quinoa. You see where I'm going with this? *Processed* can sound scary because we are told processed foods contribute to illnesses and conditions such as high blood pressure or heart diseases.

And yes, there are varying levels of processed foods. Though we are starting to use the term *ultra-processed* to describe foods like potato chips and candy bars, we still need to stop associating those foods with being bad. For starters, foods such as soy products, alternative milks, and some protein and fiber bars are also in the ultra-processed category. Those foods still provide plenty of nutrition, even with the scary name. And it's time for us to stop calling them bad. They are food items—they don't have moral value.

There are so many reasons why people choose foods that are packaged, canned, frozen, or fresh. I'm going to sound like a broken record since I brought this up in chapter four, but here are a few more ideas for you to keep in mind the next time you get worked up about processed food.

- **Affordability.** There are many different ways to include nutrient-rich foods, and people need to choose an option that fits within their budget. If that means canned or frozen, that's fine.

- **Accessibility.** Packaged foods are more widely available and also easier to manage for those with disabilities. When someone chooses the most accessible option for them, that is fine.

- **Time.** We're adults. And adults are busy. Not everyone feels like making a meal from scratch, and we often want something that saves us some time, which packaged foods do. There's nothing wrong with that.

- **Preference.** I personally love canned mandarin oranges. They're delicious, and you're not going to convince me otherwise. If you have some preferences for the packaged versions of food, that's completely fine.

So don't hate on processed foods. They are considered convenience foods, and their purpose is to be convenient. They can be so incredibly helpful for many time-strapped adults, and are a great way to add nourishment throughout the day. Getting in nutrient-rich foods is highly encouraged, but don't judge someone for how they choose to do so. Don't yuck someone else's yum.

Food for Thought 6: Diversify your plate.

I'm not just talking about eating the rainbow and getting your five servings of fruits and vegetables. I definitely try to do that, but I'm suggesting *really* diversifying your intake. This can be a tough one for those of us overcoming dieting and restriction, since we are used to limiting ourselves and only eating certain foods. If we are used to tracking every morsel and following a set list of foods we can and cannot have, we will become accustomed to one way of eating. Eating this way, we grow so familiar with the number of calories in specific foods that even if we no longer look at the label, we have internalized those allotments. That is why so many past dieters have issues trying new foods. Eating something without looking at the label or trying a dish for which you don't know every ingredient can be nerve-wracking. I get it. I've been there. But it's also so good for us. Our body needs and utilizes so many different nutrients. We tend to focus on the macros (such as carbohydrates, proteins, and fats) and fail to consider all the important micronutrients our body needs. If you eat the same foods every day, there is a slim chance you are really getting all the necessary nutrients.

I cannot emphasize enough that there shouldn't be a hierarchy of foods. Not every food is meant to provide the same nutrient or the same benefit. Some foods will provide us with iron, which is an essential mineral that helps transport oxygen from the lungs to the rest of the body—and we, of course, need plenty of oxygen in order for our muscles to function.[4] And speaking of eating a variety of foods, certain food combinations, like vitamin C–rich foods, can increase absorption. This is the case for and point of variety.

Let's look at choline, for example. Not as mainstream or sexy as, say, iron or vitamin D, but this is an essential nutrient (not a vitamin or mineral) that impacts liver function, healthy brain development, muscle movement, nervous system function, and metabolism.[5] But hardly anybody ever focuses on it. We get this nutrient from eggs, salmon, broccoli, cauliflower, liver, and more. If you are coming off a diet where you limited eggs or crucifers, you probably aren't getting enough choline. Let's look at another example—probiotics. Most people have heard of these, and there are lots of products (in food and supplement form) that promote probiotic activity. Who doesn't want a healthy gut and to poop more often, right? Listen, probiotics are great, but did you know that you also need some prebiotics, which feed your probiotics, to go along with them for the best results? Prebiotics can be found in unfermented foods such as garlic, asparagus, bananas, oats, apples, and more.

Unnecessarily limiting yourself to specific foods is really doing yourself a disservice. All foods provide something for your body. Our bodies are designed to be fueled by different nutritional components. No one single food has all the nutrition that we need. Not to mention that varying intake is also great for our microbiome, which assists with our immune system and protects us against toxins.[6]

Sometimes this can be difficult for some folks because of a dieting routine. While on a diet, we get accustomed to eating the same foods because those were the foods we were allowed. (Yes, I recognize that there are certain neurodivergent tendencies that cause people to pick the same foods because of the familiarity, but in this case, I am talking about diet culture only. Remember, I cannot cater my advice to every single person and every single situation because this is a book for the mass public, not an individual counseling session.) It is also possible to actually like the same foods from the dieting years. The difference is, what would your reaction be to change? What would your reaction be to eating something that you don't know the nutrition content of? Note that I said nutrition content, not ingredients, because yes, some of us need to know the ingredients.

Food for Thought 7: Meal planning can be your friend.

I'll let you in on a little secret: I don't like to cook. It's not my jam at all. Soon after I became an RD, I realized nourishment doesn't have to look like a perfectly curated recipe book. Meal planning can be a clever and easy way to get around this. A little trick of the trade that I like to give folks is to think about your upcoming week. Are you going to have back-to-back late work nights? Do you know that you tend to get tired of cooking once or twice a week and will probably order out? Or maybe you have a fun girls' night out or date-night plans and know you won't be cooking those days. This all counts as meal planning. It doesn't have to include hours of cutting and chopping food (it's fine if it does, of course), but it is still helpful to plan ahead.

I recommend stocking up on foods that you can quickly pre-pare. This is when having a supply of pantry items or frozen foods really comes in handy. Cans of beans that can be added to salads, helping you get in some protein and fiber, are great; you could also use cans of tuna, sardines, or chicken for bulking up a salad. Canned soups are easy to heat up. Frozen vegetables are a great economical choice if you find that you are constantly cleaning out your vegetable drawer. Grocery stores such as Trader Joe's have frozen cooked proteins like meatballs, chicken, and fish that you can easily add to dishes. Premade salads and already diced vegetables are also great fridge additions. Ready-made rice and pasta and even complete meals are great to keep on hand to get you through the week.

I know that social media makes it look as though everyone is part of a cooking competition on the Food Network, but I promise you that is not the case. Not everything on social media is real. You also have to consider that not everyone has the same circumstances as you do. Our financial situations are very different. Our grocery store access is very different. Some people have two or more children and/or are a single parent. Some people are working more than one job. We are not all in the same boat. Do what works for you individually.

Food for Thought 8: You're not always going to feel hungry; eat anyway.

Here's a hard truth: you're not always going to feel hungry, but you need to eat anyway. We are constantly being told that as a society we eat too much and overconsume food. Hence the reason why people feel the need to download apps to micromanage their intake. But so many people aren't fueling their bodies enough. We ignore our hunger cues because that's what we think we should be doing to curb our obsession, or maybe we are distracted by work, life, and stress, or are taking medication that suppresses our appetite. There's more to it than just a growling stomach to signal to us that it's time for food. Clients are often surprised at this fact, because like so many people, forgoing eating was their norm. Many people believe that they are just fine surviving on coffee in the morning. It is normal to think this way, because the volume of liquids can give us false satiety. This occurs with coffee especially, because we tend to drink it for the energy. You know what else gives us energy?

Food. So while we tend to think we need that second or third cup of coffee, we don't acknowledge that maybe what we need instead is food. We often think of the what when it comes to eating (as in the specific food), but it is also helpful to think of the how often.

I know this concept might sound confusing at first, especially since I've been repeating that you need to listen to your body. But if you're taking a medication—for instance, certain treatments for ADHD—then you may be dealing with a side effect that can suppress your normal hunger cues. In this case, your body does need its supply of calories, but you're not aware of it. The same thing can happen when we're under stress, and guess what—those are times when you really need to make sure you're eating. Here's a fun tidbit: we should aim to eat every three to four hours. This can, of course, vary with the size of your portions, but if you notice that hours have passed since you last ate, you might want to grab some food, even if you're not feeling hungry yet. Eating consistently is helpful not only for avoiding energy slumps (hello, calories) but also for balancing blood sugars.

If you are taking medications that affect your cues, try setting alarms or reminders to eat. It might seem strange to have a reminder go off that says "EAT!" but it works for some folks. In this case, your body still needs its supply of calories, but you're not aware of it. When we are attempting to meet deadlines at work and are hyperfocused, going through a traumatic time in our life, or maybe taking certain medications, eating consistently may be harder than it sounds. Not to mention that we tend to feel a growling stomach, but there are other signals that our bodies can give us when they need energy. One common signal is tiredness. Makes sense, right? Calories are units of energy, and tiredness might mean a lack of energy to some. Another sign or signal might be being hangry. Yes, that is actually a real signal. That irritability you feel when your body requires energy isn't made up. We know glucose states are low when people are hungry, and that the brain requires glucose and doesn't function properly in low-glucose states. Other common signs and signals can include shakiness or dizziness.[7]

This is where my favorite word, *nuance*, comes in. Having a non-diet approach means figuring out your body's individual needs without a restrictive mindset. In some cases, it might indeed be helpful to pay closer attention to the times of meals and also set timers, alarms, or reminders to tell you to eat.

Food for Thought 9: Cookies and yoga can coexist.

Exercise is not penance for eating. It's so wild that we normalize the rhetoric that we have to earn our food and don't deserve to eat. Eating is the very thing that keeps us alive, so no, it doesn't have to be earned.

How many articles have you seen that list a bad food in one column and then a certain exercise and duration in another column? One hot dog equals thirty minutes of Pilates. One ice cream sundae equals forty-five minutes on the treadmill. One slice of pizza equals eighty minutes of swimming. To constantly think of movement as merely calorie torching instead of associating it with all the amazing benefits it can provide—improving brain health, strengthening bones and muscles, and, very importantly, improving our ability to do everyday activities—is intensely problematic.[8]

I often find that this is the reason many people have difficulty settling on a form of movement they enjoy. Many people tend to look for the one movement activity that will burn the most calories instead of looking for something they truly enjoy. But as any rom-com fan will tell you, "Exercise gives you endorphins. Endorphins make you happy."[9] Say what you will about Elle Woods, but she wasn't entirely wrong. Exercise is linked to reducing stress by reducing levels of the stress-related hormones cortisol and adrenaline and improving mood. This is an important point to make, because if we are constantly stressed about a fitness class we are partaking in or an instructor that we find triggering, it will indeed counteract any stress-reducing benefit.

Your movement does not have to be the most expensive spin class downtown. It does not have to be the trendy barre class that all your coworkers are always talking about. It does not have to be the boot camp that takes place in a darkly lit room with an overbearing instructor. Your movement can be something that you truly love to do that makes you happy. You know the difference between happiness and dread. Yes, of course, we can want something that challenges us and leaves us dripping with sweat. However, there is still a difference between *Wow, that class was hard, and I feel amazing having gotten through it* and *Wow, that class was hard, and my body doesn't feel quite right.* Find your joy—and your joy might look different from what all the cool kids are doing.

Food for Thought 10: Fed is best.

This isn't just for babies. Everyone needs to eat, and food is a human right. It's a privilege to be able to choose from various forms of food. It's a privilege to be told to just eat the cookie because it tastes good. Some people, because of food insecurity, are thinking about how to get in their next meal. Some people are struggling with job security and have multiple mouths to feed and need a way to make their dollar stretch. I was once asked during an interview what was the key to health I could tell everyone. I simply replied "Money." Because there is no universal way to be healthy. Needless to say, that wasn't the answer they were looking for, and they finally got me to say "Eat a variety of foods," but the secret really is money.

"You're giving such a dystopian view of the world. People can access food stamps, and there are food pantries and aid that's available." I've gotten several such comments on my social media posts. Imagine thinking that the Band-Aid solutions of food pantries and food stamps to economic and societal barriers was an actual comeback to my post about recognizing privilege and the social determinants of health. And just so we're clear, the term *food stamps* isn't really used anymore; most refer to it as the Supplemental Nutrition Assistance Program (SNAP).[10] So, yes, I could easily tell this person didn't know much about public assistance and was just trying to argue for the sake of arguing. I never engage with these people, because they love arguing and negging. I refuse to waste my time and energy on those who intentionally misunderstand and misconstrue words. Food banks and SNAP don't fix problems. These programs remind me of when you lose a button from your clothing and use a safety pin temporarily. The safety pin shouldn't be used forever.

I once chatted with a teacher who was disheartened that his teenage students were eating bags of chips in the morning. He thought it was wild that these teenagers would choose that in the morning to consume. He also mentioned that the school was in a low-income neighborhood, so I did the math and offered another idea that he might not have thought about: "That might be the only thing they can afford to eat in the morning.

It might be chips or nothing." We tend to see an action as outsiders and judge accordingly. We don't realize that sometimes, to that person, that food is the better choice because it beats starving. A fifty-cent bag of chips is still providing energy. Is this an ideal meal providing a wide variety of nutrients? No, of course not, but fed is best. I want people to eat fruits, vegetables, whole grains, and proteins. I want people to feel joy when eating the cookie that they chose over the apple because they wanted something chocolatey. I want people to eat consistently and nourish their bodies with sustained energy for the day. I want people to have choices and access to those choices. But I also want people fed someway and somehow.

The above are some affirmations and thoughts to digest as a starting point to finding your own individualized way to food freedom. Your food freedom might look different from everyone else's based on your lived experience, but it doesn't mean that it's wrong. Whatever it is, it is your truth and should still be validated. In the next chapter, we will go through some scenarios, along with some helpful charts and checklists, to help you on your journey.

CHAPTER EIGHT

REFRAME YOUR APPROACH TO FOOD

Our words matter. The words we choose convey our thoughts and feelings. Aside from nonverbal communication, words are the heartbeat of our relationships.
—Mel Schwartz, LCSW[1]

Reframing our thoughts around food sounds so simple in principle. I've heard many clients and folks online say the equivalent of "Well, I'm over dieting and restricting, so now I have a neutral approach to food." But do you really? Thanks to years of diet culture, we sometimes subconsciously place food in a hierarchy. We have been programmed to think certain foods are good and others are not so good; it takes time to reframe our thoughts.

I know this firsthand. I can remember the period following my official breakup with diet culture. It was different from the "healthy" lifestyle that I had lived previously. This didn't happen when I deleted a calorie-counting app from my phone or stopped counting calories as I ate. It was years after that, when I slowly realized I wasn't to blame for my feelings around food. It wasn't me, it was diet culture, and we just weren't a good match for each other. It was only when I fully accepted this that I really embraced food neutrality and started getting excited about food again. And let me tell you, really knowing what your body needs and wants is an amazing feeling. There are times when I crave specific vegetables like Brussels sprouts or asparagus. (My six-year-old self would probably be horrified to read this.) But there are also times when I don't want any vegetables and my body asks for more protein or grains, and I am not terrified by that prospect. Our bodies won't revolt if we aren't eating picturesque meals. And there is no one food that causes disease or illness, nor is there one food that magically makes us the picture of health. For example, I eat something sweet every day, and I'm not talking about fruit. There is a container of chocolate candy in my living room and there are multiple pints of ice cream in my freezer. This probably sounds like a recipe for disaster or even like a lack of willpower, but keeping something in plain sight, viewing it as a neutral food, and giving yourself permission to have said food unconditionally is the actual food freedom recipe. Not to mention, of course, that eating all the food groups consistently helps with feeling the need to binge on sweets. There are many pieces to the puzzle of food neutrality, and acknowledging that I am wholeheartedly allowing myself to have these foods when I want is helpful. Yes, it is easier said than done, but rebuilding a positive relationship with food doesn't happen overnight. The more I allow myself to have these things, the less I fear them or feel as though I can't control myself. I don't view sweets as treats or sometime foods or even as bad. They are sweet-tasting foods that I enjoy when I have a taste for them. Because of this mentality I can have a few pieces and be satisfied. And sometimes I have more than a few pieces.

There's no universal serving size that applies to every individual or every occasion.

A major part of my own recovery involved reframing how I viewed food. I recognize how hard this is, so this is something I work on with all my clients, no matter what their concerns are. I can't even count how many times people have come to me with a preconceived idea of what working on a healthy relationship with food entails. Thanks to diet culture, there is a desire to prove how healthy one can eat or how many nutrient-dense meals one can make during the week. There is nothing wrong with wanting to improve your physical health, but we have to first acknowledge that

- Health is individual and subjective.

- Health is more than what we eat and how much we exercise.

- There are systemic barriers to getting healthy in place for some.

Without understanding and accepting these three principles, your journey toward health won't be sustainable.

An extremely important part of healthy eating is knowing that different foods are going to give us different nutrients and attributes. This means that a chocolate chip cookie can be equated to a salad in some instances because both foods can actually decrease our stress levels regarding food, which is health promoting. That is the heart of food neutrality.

I know that some of you may have read that last paragraph in disbelief, but it's true. Food is a neutral entity, neither good nor bad. In an article from *Psychology Today*, Jeremy Shapiro, PhD, discusses why we tend to have such black-and-white views: "In polarized thinking, people typically seize on one pole of a spectrum as purely good and reject the other pole as purely bad, and they become fixated on one extreme point of view to the exclusion of all other perspectives. This cognitive style prevents people from being aware of the full range of possibilities available to them. People feel they must make either/or choices when there are actually many options in between."[2]

That is exactly how I would describe our way of thinking around food and eating. If there is a "good" food, there must be a "bad" food. But that's just not the case.

• SO YOU'RE OVER DIETING— • OKAY, NOW WHAT?

An important step is to reframe our approach to food. Food is eaten not just for its nutrients and it is not representative of our moral value as humans. Here is how we think we choose food:

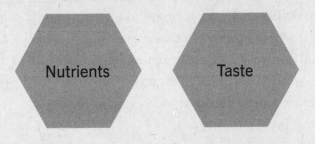

But in reality, there are many factors, and our choices look something like this:

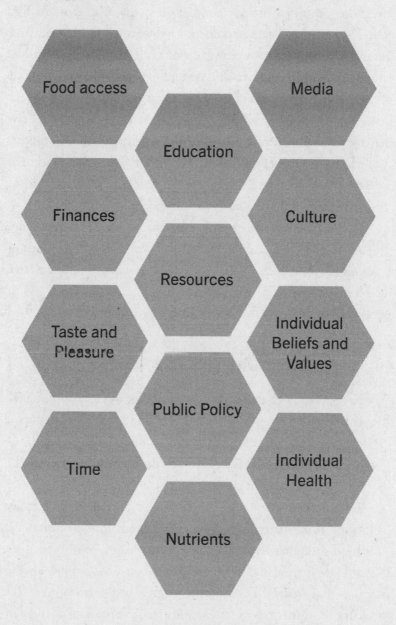

There are many factors that go into our food choices because we are complex individuals. We are told to base most of our food decisions around nutrient content, but that isn't sustainable. There are personal factors affecting why we choose foods, and many of those factors are out of our control. Not to mention, of course, that it's okay to choose and eat foods that taste good. Even in this chapter, I'm talking about reframing—without a name or label—your whole approach to eating. The very existence of a label makes it seem like there must be rules to follow. I like to think of it as figuring out a way of eating that works for you that will not take a toll on your physical and mental health. It doesn't have to have a name or a category.

As you dive into this new approach, remember that *you* are the one in charge. *You* are figuring out a way to consume foods in a way that works for *you*—a way that is joyful and not restrictive and allows a sense of mental freedom.

• THE WORDS WE USE MATTER •

We have become so accustomed to assigning adjectives that have either a negative or a positive connotation to food. For example, "This is my cheat meal of the week." "This cake is so sinful." "I feel so guilty whenever I order the fries instead of the salad." Sound familiar? I could go on and on.

Reframing our words is such an important approach to really achieving food neutrality. These words seem innocent enough, but food shouldn't have negative connotations. Food is neutral. What if we instead described food by what it tastes like? Or the textures that we feel? For example, eggs Benedict isn't a treat. It's a savory meal that has a rich, creamy hollandaise sauce (and I'm going to assume it's delicious). And on the other end, your salad isn't a good meal. (I know that you're thinking *Wait, what?* Yes. When you stop categorizing food, no food is called good or bad.)

And why not call more foods good? Because if you label something good, that means something else has to be labeled bad, and that's when we feel bad or stressed even for eating. A salad might provide nutrients such as vitamins A, C, E, and K, and perhaps more fiber will keep your tummy fuller and your digestive system more regular; that's great, yes, but it doesn't place it at the top of a moral hierarchy. French fries provide nutrients like vitamins C and B_6, as well as the mineral potassium, even though they are fried. Do I suggest living off fries? No. But guess what: I don't suggest only eating salads either. There is a place for both. (I mean, I have definitely ordered a salad because I wanted something crunchy and cold with some sweet and/or tart taste notes, but I also wanted fries—especially if they are steak cut—and decided to get that, too.)

A quick grammar lesson here to illustrate. Let's break down this popular phrase:

This is my cheat meal because I was so good all week.

And now let's focus on specific words:

This is my **cheat meal** because I was so good all week.

Cheat (noun)—the act or an instance of fraudulently deceiving.

Cheat (verb)—to deprive of something valuable by the use of deceit or fraud.[3]

Here, *cheat* is being used as an adjective to describe your meal. If we look at the various definitions of *cheat*, they are negative, mostly associated with being fraudulent or deceitful.

This is my cheat meal because I was **so good** all week.

Good (noun)—virtuous, right, commendable.[4]

You are using *good* to describe yourself, and you are equating yourself with a certain moral value.

This might seem a bit extra, but we need to start realizing that words matter, and how we use words to talk about ourselves matters. We are equating the foods that we eat with our values or our character. That should never be the case.

Negative descriptors include the following:

- Toxic

- Treat

- Cheat meal

- Junk

- Sinful

- Bad

- Good

- Guilty pleasure

- Guilt-free

- Problem

- Garbage

- Addictive

- Forbidden

I urge you to try to strip these words from your vocabulary when referring to food. When I work with clients, I ask them to really try to describe the food on their plate. I think of the preschoolers that I work with and how we teach them to use their five senses. As adults, it wouldn't hurt for us to try this for ourselves.

Next time you sit down to a meal, before taking a bite, really look at the food in front of you. Try to think about and describe the following:

- **Sight:** Note the colors you are seeing and the plating of the food. The colors might be dull instead of vibrant, which can be a turnoff. Or the foods might all run into one another.

- **Smell:** Smell plays a huge role in what we consider appetizing. Think of the freshly baked croissant or the garlic roasted vegetables in the oven. Our mouths may begin salivating at the very thought.

- **Sound:** Yes, sound. The sound of the crunch that happens when you bite into a French fry or when your spoon digs into the top layer of a crème brûlée.

- **Touch:** Think of all the foods that we eat with our hands. Better yet, think of all the different cultural cuisines that are consumed sans silverware. Make notes of the food being soft or hard.

- **Taste:** And, finally, describe the taste. We have taste buds for a reason, so make note of what they are telling you.

Those latter two categories are the most important as we begin trying to describe food differently. Here are some descriptors we can start using:

For touch:

- Hard

- Soft

- Creamy

- Hot

- Cold

- Thick

- Fuzzy

- Prickly

- Flaky

- Smooth

And for taste:

- Sweet

- Salty

- Savory

- Bland

- Tart

- Sour

- Bitter

- Buttery

- Spicy

- Unseasoned

When we use certain words, we internalize messages about food, whether we are cognizant of it or not. Positive words encourage brain function, while negative words activate our fight-or-flight response, which slows cognitive function. As Dr. Andrew Newberg, a neuroscientist who studies the relationship between brain function and various mental states, writes in *Words Can Change Your Brain*, "A single word has the power to influence the expression of genes that regulate physical and emotional stress."[5] It's the idea that practicing positive thinking can reduce heart rate and help us with anxiety. Negative words, on the flip side, trigger fear and generate internal stress in the body and a feeling of hopelessness. As a result, they adversely affect motivation.

All of this is honestly a fancy way of saying that our adjectives matter. The words we attach to food to describe them are not just innocent throwaway sentences that you might say over brunch with friends. They can, in fact, impact how we feel about ourselves. This is why learning to use different descriptors is so important when it comes to reframing our thoughts.

And that isn't easy. It took us time to learn these thought patterns, and so it takes time to reframe them.

With that, let's try another set, using feelings around ice cream as a test case:

I'm so bad for craving this ice cream.
I'm so bad for craving this ice cream.

We are not bad people for wanting ice cream. Sure, ice cream isn't the same as a vegetable, but no one is saying these foods are the same—so stop calling yourself bad for wanting it. If it is a hot summer afternoon and we have been outside all day, sometimes our bodies are asking for something sweet, cold, and creamy. We are not bad people for wanting a certain food.

I'm so bad for craving this **ice cream**.

Ice cream is just a certain type of food. It is a sweet, cold, and creamy food, but not a bad food. What can make it bad? Ice cream is only bad if it's not sweet enough for you, or the flavor is not great, or if it is melting because it's not cold anymore. It's not inherently bad. But even that is based on individual preferences, as we all have different taste buds. So the ice cream isn't a bad food—just the taste of it can be. Try articulating that instead. We can use actual adjectives and descriptors related to our senses to describe what we are eating.

And some more:

Instead of "That meal did not cut it. That was such a waste of calories! I'm never ordering that again."

Reframe with "That meal did not cut it. That was a waste for my taste buds and my wallet. I'm never ordering that and wasting my money again."

We are 100 percent allowed to not enjoy our food because of taste or some other personal preference. However, we tend to attach what we don't like to diet culture through our word choices. The diet mentality still associates calories with something to be avoided. For instance, the phrase "waste of calories" implies that we're restricting our caloric intake and that we should feel guilty about eating. Even though we didn't enjoy the meal, it was still providing nutrients and energy for our body to use. It wasn't a waste—it just wasn't as tasty as we'd hoped. Reframing our thoughts can still imply that this meal sucked and would not get the best Yelp review, but it comes without the side of diet culture and restriction.

• ALL-OR-NOTHING THINKING •

As humans, we tend to see everything in binaries: good or bad, success or failure, all or nothing. So when trying to rebuild your relationship with food and finding a method of eating that works for you, you might feel discouraged by setbacks, especially when the bar is set to perfection. I've had many clients tell me "I'll never get to food neutrality" because a couple of times they ate past fullness and had an uncomfortable feeling afterward, which they equated with failure. But when we approach it with that mindset, we are discounting the positive, ignoring the times we ate with contentment and satisfaction. We get frustrated with our choices, so we decide that food neutrality will never happen and that our relationship won't improve. Not to be too blasé about it, but that is all in our heads.

Cognitive distortion can be described as internal mental filters or biases that increase our misery, fuel our anxiety, and make us feel bad about ourselves.[6] And when it comes to eating, becoming aware of your cognitive distortions can help you reframe them and find your way back to eating with joy and freedom.

Notice the distortion. For example, if you're adding more dressing to a dry salad, check in and see if you're feeling guilty or "gross." Are you telling yourself that this dressing is making the salad unhealthy? Are you thinking that you've failed at yet another diet simply by making your salad taste better? Try the following:

- **Evaluate the evidence:** Remove your thoughts and emotions for a second and think about what the actual facts of the situation are. Can you reframe it? The facts are, you're eating a salad that is full of vitamins, fiber, and phytonutrients. By adding dressing, you are adding fats, which your body requires, as fat helps us absorb the vitamins A, D, E, and K, which can be found in certain ingredients in the salad. You are also adding an acid (likely lemon juice or vinegar), which can serve as an antioxidant. More importantly, you are also making the salad taste good, which means you will not only eat it but you will also *enjoy* it.

- **Practice compassion:** Do not expect perfection from yourself. Do not expect yourself to eat a handful of raw kale when you don't want to. Part of having a great relationship with food is to fully grant yourself permission to find joy in your food. Remember, one meal, one day of food choices, or even a few days of food choices doesn't make you a bad person. There is no timeline. We must work on learning to bounce back from this mentality and know it's okay to eat a variety of foods.

Reframing our thoughts can take time, especially when we're so used to placing things in categories. It also takes time to not plate check or body check others. We often look at others around us to influence our choices. But in these times, it's vital to remember that it's your body, your needs, and your wants. Whatever someone else is eating, that's fine for them. It's okay to want something different. For instance, your friend is ordering the BLT sandwich with a salad, but you have been thinking about fries for a few days. Instead of just having them and moving on, you second-guess yourself: *Should I also order the salad? The salad is healthier. I don't want to look bad eating fries.*

You are your own individual person, and once again, food should not be put in a hierarchy. We think of salad as a good food and fries as a bad food. But with the mindset of food neutrality, we would know that fries and salad are just two different foods providing two different tastes and two different sets of nutrients. That's all.

• EAT WHEN YOU'RE HUNGRY •

Practicing food neutrality takes some time to get used to, which is normal. Nothing happens overnight. Along with attaching a moral compass to food, we also constantly convince ourselves that we shouldn't eat and that being hungry is wrong. Food is necessary for our bodies, and it is a human right. So this will be a reminder from your friendly dietitian: if you're hungry, you should eat something.

Thanks to diet culture, we too often put our hunger on the back burner. Even when we do acknowledge our hunger, we come up with reasons why we shouldn't eat. *I just ate; I can't possibly be hungry. I had such a large meal beforehand; I shouldn't be hungry already.* Don't deny hunger. Eating is a perfectly natural, very human act. There are going to be times when we get busy and food isn't always readily available, or we might have a condition or take medication that throws off our hunger cues. This is different than intentionally denying our hunger because of diet culture. I also have to add here that coffee is great in the morning, but that's not breakfast. It's coffee. It's a liquid that gives us temporary volume so we feel full, but we're not really, and it would be great to eat something with your morning cup of caffeinated goodness. Adding to that, gum is something to freshen your breath with. So many resources on dieting and how to put off hunger list gum as a good way to trick your body into thinking that you're eating. And, finally, that fancy green juice that costs fifteen dollars is a drink *with* your meal—it's definitely not a meal in itself.

• REMEMBERING TO EAT •

There may be occasions when you get really busy and life gets in the way, and all of a sudden you go, *Wow, I forgot to eat.* Our bodies are pretty amazing at signaling their needs (growling stomachs, for instance) but stress, medications, and neurodivergent conditions such as ADHD can suppress those cues. There are some tips for figuring out whether or not you really are hungry.

I highly recommend checking in on yourself and noticing when your body is signaling that it needs food. Your body needs different amounts and types of food on different days. Honor that need.

When was the last time you ate?

More than three hours ago   **Less than three hours ago**

Still check in   **Still check in**

Note any physical signals

Stomach Growls
Headache
Low Energy
Lightheadedness
Stomach Cramping/Pain
Moodiness or Irritability

To do so, I want you to start asking yourselves:

1. When was my last meal? How many hours have passed since I last ate?

   If you have trouble believing that you're hungry, think about whether the last thing you ate contained the trifecta of carbohydrates, protein, and fat. This is what helps sustain us. If this still checks, ask whether you are moving your body, requiring more energy. If the answer is no, you can still be hungry because your biological and metabolic needs change daily.

   Ask, what sensations am I feeling in my body? Choose one of the options below in each pairing.

   • Alert or distracted
   • Tired or energetic
   • Irritable or neutral

2. What foods are accessible? Access to food plays a huge role in how we eat and whether we are able to do it consistently. Recall that fed is best. I am also a fan of having snacks readily available if possible so when the hunger pang hits, you can satisfy it.

Still not feeling it? Literally or figuratively? This is when my favorite word, *nuance*, comes into play. While, generally speaking, I'm not a fan of external cues and permission to eat via dieting apps and rules, sometimes we need external cues to help us, like when stress, medications, and neurodivergent tendencies play a role in our hunger.

Here are some suggestions for a helping hand:

- Set an alarm or a timer. When we're busy and in the zone with work, time gets ahead of us. Setting an alarm or a timer for three or four hours after your first meal to remind you to eat might be helpful.

- Schedule meals. Put "eat lunch" on your calendar for 12:00 p.m. so you get an alert. I'm serious.

- Keep accessible snacks close. The more hyperfocused we are, the less likely we will stop what we are doing for something as annoying as eating. **Insert winking emoji.** I'm the queen of snacks, a title I gave to myself because my friends make fun of me for carrying food around all the time—and I mean all the time. I also keep snacks handy in a drawer in my office cubicle. These are nonperishable snacks that I actually enjoy and will eat.

If you're not sure what snacks might work for you, here are some of my friendly suggestions and personal nonperishable (desk- and drawer-friendly) favorites:

- Individual nut butter packets

- Container of nuts

- Packets of dried fruit

- Dried edamame

- Pretzels (the ones filled with peanut/almond butter can also be good)

- Beef/turkey jerky

- Popcorn

- Whole-grain tortilla chips

- Protein bars

- Fiber bars

Want to get a bit fancier? Try making your own trail mix:

- 1 part cereal (Cheerios, Chex, Shredded Wheat, whatever you're feeling)

- 1 part nuts or seeds (such as sunflower or pumpkin) or both

- 1 part dried fruit (cranberries, cherries, or blueberries)

- Yes, you can also add those M&M's or chocolate chips if you want

Sometimes we put off eating because food and choices are overwhelming. Take that choice overload away with some of the following snacks and quick-grab meals:

- Prepackaged fiber and protein bars

- Individualized containers of yogurt

- Individualized containers of cottage cheese

- Packaged nut mix with dried fruit

- Toast with cream cheese or nut butter spread

- Frozen waffles spread with yogurt, nut butter, and/or fruit

- Packaged instant oatmeal

- Hummus with whole-grain crackers or vegetables

- Dry cereal in a reusable plastic bag

- Individualized bottles of kefir or drinkable yogurt

- PB&J sandwich (or substitute any other nut butter)

- Cereal with milk

- Smoothies (try to add proteins like yogurt, nut butter, or protein powders)

- Deli meat with cheese and crackers (mini charcuterie)

- Sandwich wraps

- Boiled eggs (can be made in a batch for the week)

• QUICK MEALS FOR BUSY ADULTS •

On my TikTok channel, I started a series called *Quick Meals for Busy Adults*. It started as a joke because I feel that social media is so carefully curated and pretty. We see these influencers in their beautiful, spotless kitchens with amazing lighting and organized spice racks. That's all fine and good, but some of us are schlepping home after a long day of work. We're in our sweatpants, bonnets, and messy buns trying to feed ourselves. We are not all pretty and curated. So, there I was in my poorly lit kitchen after work, determined to show what many adults actually look like when cooking. That first video took off, followers started asking for more of that content, and now here we are. So here are some of my favorite quick meals:

- Prepackaged salad of your choice—saves time with not having to chop; it's easy to open, and as simple to

prepare as pouring it into a large bowl. If I have nuts
and dried fruit on hand, I add that as well.

- Tinned fish—sardines, tuna, salmon. Easy to open and
  can be added to salads and used in sandwiches. Great
  protein option and a way to get in those omega-3s.

- Rotisserie chicken—this is such a lifesaver for a quick
  protein option. Many grocery stores have them, and
  they can be used as a meal's main protein option or
  added to salads or pastas.

- Frozen ready-made chicken cutlets, strips, nuggets (yes,
  nuggets, even if you don't have kids)—another great
  protein option to have on hand when you haven't gone
  grocery shopping. I love frozen options that are quick
  and easy to pop in the oven or on the stove.

- Chicken sausage—another protein option. I like adding this to rice dishes especially. It is also a yummy option for breakfast with eggs.

- Can of beans—protein and fiber packed in one. Use in
  rice and beans or add to pasta dishes, salads, or baked
  potatoes. (Don't knock it until you try it!)

- Frozen vegetables—as I mentioned before, I love frozen
  options. Fresh produce has a tendency to go bad in the
  refrigerator because we forget about it. Frozen veggies
  last longer, and the produce is picked and frozen at ripe-
  ness, which means you are still getting the nutrients.

- Frozen fruit—same as its frozen vegetable counterparts
  and can be added in smoothies or eaten as is.

- Russet potatoes—poke some holes and stick them in the microwave for a "baked" potato.

- One-minute rice—a great way to get your grains. There are so many quick options, and some are flavored. One of my favorites is a yellow rice option; add chicken sausage and some veggies.

- Pasta—pretty quick to make with some store-bought sauce. Also, if you have leftover pasta, don't throw it away! Save it to use for cold pasta salads.

- Tortilla wraps—serve as the outer layer of quesadillas or sandwich wraps. Stuff with your choice of protein and vegetables.

• FOOD ALLERGIES •

I'm allergic to nuts, soy, and green peas, and it kind of sucks. Not to mention there are foods I'm intolerant of that make my stomach hurt. Trust me, it feels like a betrayal, to be intolerant of avocado and pineapple as a dietitian. It's annoying to have to constantly look at the ingredient list or be *that* person who is grilling the waiter about the items on the menu. You feel like you can never truly have the freedom that others do, because you know the slightest mix-up can be dangerous or leave you feeling uncomfortable. I get it.

For some reason, the fact that I have food allergies surprises people on social media. People always seem to believe that dietitians are perfect when it comes to food. But that's just plain false. I have some food allergies, and I also have some health issues because I'm human. In fact, many dietitians will tell you that having food allergies is part of why they got into the field: to help others just like them. So yes, there are foods that I enjoy and there are foods that I cannot eat freely. This does *not* take away from the all-foods-can-fit mentality. If something doesn't agree with your body, then don't eat it. It's actually that simple. I feel neutral when I go out to Mexican restaurants with friends and am the only one who isn't enjoying the guacamole, because my body won't let me. In my mind it's an item that I can't have . . . so I go to town on the chips and salsa instead.

I understand the frustration and annoyance of allergies. They suck, and I am 100 percent jealous of people who can throw any interesting food into their shopping cart without question or those who can vacation in other countries and just try whatever the cultural cuisine is without really knowing the ingredients. Trying to explain to people in stores and restaurants that you can't have certain ingredients in a language you don't understand will humble you really quick. But despite all of this, I acknowledge the various food options I do have.

Allergies and intolerances aren't fun, and they also contribute to the hows and whys of eating. If we look into our personal food history, we can see that allergies can sometimes trigger past disordered eating thoughts. We avoid foods that are going to send us into anaphylactic shock, but the feeling might bring back the triggers of food restriction from diet culture. Reflect on these feelings. Make a list of the foods that you are allergic to. Now make a list of the foods that you avoid, despite not being intolerant of them. Why are you avoiding the foods in the second category? What is triggering this fear surrounding eating them?

I will say this on repeat: the only foods you have to avoid are the ones you're allergic or intolerant to, the ones you don't like, and the ones that you can't have for medical reasons (this requires so much nuance and doesn't have to be as restrictive as some people make it).

• GETTING THAT DOPAMINE HIT •

There are indeed times when we eat that have nothing to do with hunger. Part of reframing our relationship to food is knowing that we are not morally wrong for emotionally eating, and willpower has nothing to do with any of it. We can be excited, stressed, and/or bored and want some feel-good comfort right then and there. Many of us look for this feel-goodness in the form of food when we are going through emotions. We want that hit of dopamine, a feel-good neurotransmitter our brain releases when we engage in activities like eating certain foods or having sex, which contribute to our feelings of pleasure and satisfaction as part of the reward system.[7]

Emotional eating isn't just for when we are stressed but can also be caused by, but not limited to, boredom, excitement, and sadness. Eating while feeling these emotions doesn't make you bad, and it doesn't have to be looked at as a lack of willpower. We are reframing here, and that is one of the important steps in how we view food. We can acknowledge our emotions and also start to realize when we are using food as a coping mechanism for something. We make emotional eating sound like such a horror, but we also live in a society where we are taught to view food as good or bad, so that isn't surprising. Food tastes good and can give us that dopamine hit that our body is asking for sometimes. Instead of beating ourselves up about it, we can find additional tools we can add to our toolbox for times when we are going through normal human emotions. What I'm saying is, have your cookie and the ability to choose something else that feels good, too. Some additional tools for your toolbox of dopamine hits can be the following:

- Meditation

- Yoga

- Getting a massage

- Playing with a pet

- Taking a walk outside

- Reading a book

- Knitting

- Doing jigsaw puzzles

- Painting with watercolors

- Talking with a therapist

- Using Play-Doh

- Dancing like no one's watching

- Doing crossword puzzles

- Listening to music

- Coloring in coloring books

- Scrapbooking

- Taking a bubble bath

- Talking with a friend

- Painting your nails

- Doing a DIY face mask

Eating food is not wrong—I need to emphasize this. However, I do believe in digging deeper and finding meanings behind why we might be doing something. Sometimes it is out of habit, because there are foods that just do the trick. On a hot summer day when I am feeling particularly excited, there is nothing like a good stroll outdoors *and* ice cream. There are times when I feel a heaviness in my heart because I am still grieving a loss. Watching a good movie *and* eating a dessert helps. I am not counseling each of you reading this personally, and I cannot say when the perfect time to eat for comfort is and when it might be a better idea to dig deeper and find other tools, because we are individuals and not everything can easily be explained in a book. So trust yourself, look out for binary thinking, take a step back, and think about your actions and acknowledge them.

CHAPTER NINE

TOOLS FOR YOUR TOOLBOX

I have not failed. I've just found ten thousand ways that won't work.

—Thomas A. Edison[1]

· STARTING SMALL ·

To begin working toward food freedom, the first step we can take is to list some behavior changes and slowly work them into our routine. I'm talking about starting with *one* of the below and working your way up.

Choose your goal for the week:

- Eat an extra serving of vegetables

- Eat an extra serving of fruit

- Go to bed half an hour earlier

- Take a five-minute stretch break every hour at your desk

- Drink an extra cup of water

- Don't look at any screen for a total of fifteen minutes (this is harder than it sounds)

SIDE DISCUSSION

"I don't eat vegetables."

Are you sure? Are you only considering green vegetables real vegetables? I find that when I hear this from folks, they are talking about the popular vegetables (kale, broccoli, Brussels sprouts).

These greens are not the only veggies! Here are a couple of often forgotten but still mighty veggies:

Onions—YES, onions. High in vitamins B and C, potassium, and antioxidants, and they are a prebiotic food, which is great for digestive health.

Garlic—contains vitamins B and C, manganese, and antioxidants.

Shallots—contain protein, fiber, calcium, iron, magnesium, phosphorus, potassium, zinc, copper, folate, B vitamins, and vitamins A and C.

Do not wait to sleep until you're dead.

This is one behavior that I am constantly trying to improve. Why is getting in those *z*'s so important? During sleep, your body is working to support healthy brain function and maintain your physical health. Getting inadequate sleep over time can raise your risk for chronic health problems. Lack of sleep also affects how well you think, react, work, learn, and get along with others. So, no, unlike that infamous saying, we shouldn't just wait until we're dead to sleep. Let's work on it now.

Sleep health checklist:

- Aim for at least seven hours per night. According to the Sleep Foundation, adults aged eighteen to sixty-four years need seven to nine hours. Older adults need seven to eight hours.[2]

- Set a realistic bedtime. We all don't have to be under the covers by 9:00 p.m., but take a look at your schedule and when you would need to be in bed in order to get a good seven hours of sleep.

- Limit caffeine six to eight hours before bedtime. Chamomile and lavender tea are some great soothing options for a nighttime drink.

- Limit alcohol altogether and *large* meals a few hours beforehand. (Some snacks before bedtime can be good and sleep promoting.)

- Limit screen time two hours before bed. The blue-light exposure tricks our body into thinking that it is still daytime. I'm a fan of the app f.lux (not sponsored) that works on laptops and on computers. I personally love that the app adapts the color of your computer's display to the time of day (warm at night and sunlight during the day), which can reduce strain on your eyes and promote sleep, since our screens are mostly bright.

- Take a relaxing bath or shower.

- Get comfy with the temperature, your mattress, bedsheets, and pillows.

- Use a melatonin supplement if needed. (Please consult your doctor first.)

Foods that promote sleep:

- Almonds—a source of melatonin

- Tart cherry juice—contains high levels of melatonin

- Kiwis—a great source of serotonin

- Fatty fish—the combination of omega-3 fatty acids and vitamin D in fatty fish has the potential to enhance sleep quality, as both have been shown to increase the production of serotonin

- Turkey—a source of tryptophan, which is used to make serotonin. When tryptophan makes serotonin, the byproduct is melatonin, our beloved friend and sleep regulator.

- Dairy products—also a source of tryptophan

If you find that stress from the week has been keeping you up at night, it might be helpful to write it out:

_____

_____

_____

_____

_____

What can we do about it:

- Schedule a session with a therapist.

- Go on a coffee date with a friend and tell them beforehand if you want to vent *or* if you want advice.

- If you have a safe space to do so, go on a walk to get some fresh air.

- Watch an entertaining but mindless television show. (My personal favorites are *Real Housewives*, *The Bachelor*, and *Love Is Blind*. You can obviously choose whatever you want!)

- Start journaling.

- Read a book.

Are you cranky or are you dehydrated?

Staying hydrated is so important to us all. Drinking water can prevent dehydration, which can cause confusion, mood change, body overheating, constipation, and kidney stones.

Signs of dehydration:

- Extreme thirst

- Less frequent urination

- Dark-colored urine

- Fatigue

- Dizziness

- Confusion

Make sure to increase water intake when you are

- In hot climates

- More physically active

- Running a fever

- Experiencing diarrhea or vomiting

Ways to up your daily hydration:

- Add frozen fruit, cucumber, and/or herbs to water for taste

- Keep a water bottle handy for easy access (it does not have to be an expensive one)

- Set a timer as a reminder

- Use a hydration tracking app

- Drink water before your morning coffee and/or tea, before your afternoon drink with lunch, and before your dinner drink

- Eat foods with high water content, such as cucumbers, watermelon, tomatoes, melons, and lettuce

You are allowed to eat food that tastes good and that you enjoy.

Food is one of humanity's basic needs for survival. We of course wouldn't know that given all of the media rhetoric we see on how to trick our bodies into thinking they're full. We seem to always reach for supplements (nothing wrong with some, but they are not all created equal), meal replacement shakes, or other concoctions instead of acknowledging that food contains essential nutrients our body uses for growth, repair, and maintenance of tissues and the regulation of vital processes. Food also provides the energy our bodies need to function.

Your body deserves nourishment always.

During 2020, the ongoing events definitely affected my stress levels, which in turn affected my appetite. It was one of those rare instances when I had to constantly remind myself to eat, to nourish my body properly. In times like that, listening to internal hunger cues isn't always easy, and different circumstances will require different methods. Form a routine of eating every three to four hours until your body starts to regulate again, and try some of the following.

This is a generalized list of examples *only*:

- 8:00 a.m. Breakfast—quick grabs include cereal, individual yogurt containers, toast with nut butter, oatmeal packets, frozen waffles with nut butter or yogurt, individual cottage cheese containers

- 11:00 a.m. Snack—string cheese and fruit, string cheese and crackers, trail mix, beef jerky and nuts, fiber bars, apple with nut butter, hummus with crackers, peppers, tortilla chips, or cucumbers

- 1:00 p.m. Lunch—leftovers if you cooked, cans or packets of tuna, pre-bagged salads, nut butter and jelly sandwiches, premade soups, deli meat with crackers and cucumbers

- 4:00 p.m. Snack—see morning snack above

- 7:00 p.m. Dinner—takeout, frozen dinner, cold cereal (I'm not joking), pasta with jarred sauce, make your own charcuterie, pre-bagged salads

Eat consistently, and remember: fed is best, for everyone.

You are allowed to eat food that tastes good.

I can firmly say that we have taste buds for a reason. It is one of the simplest yet also most necessary reminders that I often give people. Diet culture tells us that if we enjoy food too much, that's a problem. It's such a shame, because we really have lost the joy of eating. When steeped in diet culture, we are so focused on nutrients and what each food does for us biologically, but that should in no way be the final say. Food is meant to be enjoyable and social. There is nothing wrong with this.

One of my clients was, in her words, "bored with food." And I'm not talking the "I hate to cook and don't want to think" mentality; this was an "I eat the same thing every day and am bored, but I am scared to stray from what I know" mentality. "What was the last food you ate that excited you?" I asked, and there was about a one-minute pause. After that, she finally recalled a holiday dinner at her grandmother's that was filled with delicious food. "But it was all bad food, so I don't eat like that often." "Well, what made it bad?" "It tasted delicious, so I know that it wasn't healthy." And, boom, there it was. The feeling that so many people have of trying to serve penance for eating delicious food.

Here's how can we work through this:

Remembering that eating can be a joyous occasion and that food is associated with many joyous social interactions can be helpful, because we often think of food only as a way to provide nutrients. The social aspect of eating is so important because socialization decreases stress, and we know how much stress can affect our digestion and gut health. Associating food with joy is important.

Recall your favorite food memory:

_____

_____

_____

_____

_____

_____

_____

_____

_____

You're intrigued by the bakery you pass by with the flaky croissants, or you're curious about the jar of chili oil you're not sure what to do with but looks intriguing or the box of flavored pasta you have been eyeing because the shape just looks fun. We sometimes get into a rut with food because we are drawn to foods we ate when we were in the grasp of diet culture or we stick to what we are used to out of habit. It's a good idea to try new foods that are enticing and interesting to get us excited again. What are some foods that you've been scoping out?

_____

_____

_____

_____

_____

_____

_____

• BEYOND SALT AND PEPPER •

Do you not like a certain food, or was it just not seasoned properly? I hear adults say all the time that they force themselves to eat vegetables. Now, there is nothing wrong with taste preferences, but I do question when food groups as a whole are despised. Especially vegetables. Far too often I realize that it isn't so much the food but the way it's prepared. Are we still remembering our parents boiling and steaming vegetables without putting anything on them? Are we still thinking about saving calories by not using fats like butter or oil? I highly recommend roasting and adding flavor. This is coming from someone who doesn't like to cook but knows what tastes good.

My favorite selections:

- Cinnamon pairs well with allspice, cardamom, chili, cloves, coriander, cumin, ginger, nutmeg, and turmeric.

- Garlic pairs well with fennel seeds, oregano, parsley, pepper, rosemary, sage, tarragon, thyme, and mint.

- Ginger pairs well with cloves, coriander, cumin, fennel seed, paprika, and turmeric.

Your cultural foods are relevant.

Your cultural foods are an important tie to your heritage and background, and you can celebrate this and also eat in a way that nourishes you. Healthy eating and eating cultural foods do not cancel each other out. We as a society have a tendency to put Westernized foods on a pedestal while othering foods from different cultures. Because of societal norms, the foods that

QUICK HISTORY LESSON

Avoid unseasoned food—I'm not joking. Spice and flavor are used to enhance the taste of many dishes, not to mention that they can be beneficial for health. For example, ginger adds a nice spicy kick and is great in stir-fried dishes, juices, teas, dressings, and sweets. At the same time, ginger is also great for digestive issues, nausea, and stomach pain. Garlic, which is potent yet absolutely delicious, is great for roasted vegetables and meats, pasta sauces, soups, and stews. Further, garlic is beneficial for immune support.

I've seen several high-profile influencers post something to the effect that seasoning food is unhealthy. This is comical and also seriously untrue. It also belies the complicated history between spices and elitism.

CliffsNotes: Spices were once extremely expensive in mid-1600s Europe, which meant only the wealthy could afford to use them. However, as countries like India were colonized, spices became more readily available, more affordable, and no longer exclusive. "So the elite recoiled from the increasing popularity of spices," says Krishnendu Ray, a professor of food studies at New York University. "They moved on to an aesthetic theory of taste. Rather than infusing food with spice, they said things should taste like themselves. Meat should taste like meat, and anything you add should only serve to intensify the existing flavors."[3]

This history of spices is reminiscent of some of our wellness trends today. Many products are in limited supply, and thus are more expensive and more desirable. The less attainable something is, the more attractive it becomes.

are most often hailed as healthy are those confirmed by Western standards. This leaves many from other cultures feeling as though their foods are inferior. In health and wellness spaces, when BIPOC folks see our cultural foods represented, they're on the "red list" of foods in diet programs or they are monetized for profit, driving up costs (avocados and chia seeds).

In a mixed-methods study, twenty-four Mexican American women were interviewed about ethnic identity and its relation to the perception of health and nutrition. Although the women recognized certain Mexican foods as traditional and important to maintaining a sense of ethnic identity, they described most of these foods as unhealthy. "Whereas 'American' food was sometimes characterized as unhealthy, such as hamburgers or lasagna, and sometimes healthier, such as salads, grilled chicken, or sandwiches, Mexican foods were nearly always described as unhealthy."[4]

Growing up, I remember my dad constantly eating avocados, even in the '90s when they weren't popular and thought to be too fattening. But he would never think of parting with his beloved pear (what Jamaicans call avocado). Fast forward to the 2010s and my dad complaining about not only the lack of good pears but the cost of them. As society realized the amazing health benefits, the pear, or avocado, that is a staple of many cultural cuisines was deemed a superfood.

I repeat the above example constantly because I have heard from so many BIPOC folks that their foods aren't healthy, that they need to healthify their cuisines even though they aren't exactly sure why. Every culture has foods filled with nutrients that are beneficial to us. No culture is superior to any other, because foods are eaten according to region, the lifestyle of that region, the holidays and celebrations of that region, and much more. I also notice that our society tends to associate some cultures with eating fewer vegetables. But in actuality, all cultures eat vegetables, just differently. Salsas, soups, broths, stews, sautés, and drinks can all contain vegetables, and we still get nutrients from them.

Your cultural foods aren't unhealthy or in need of fixing. As an individual, you might need to focus on altering one or two ingredients in a dish, but that is vastly different from classifying a culture as a whole as unhealthy. Remember: embracing your cultural foods is the greatest form of resistance against a society that's constantly asking you to change how you eat and to assimilate.

We don't have to connect food with exercise.

I have always had a complicated relationship with movement. As someone who is hyperactive and in constant need of stimulation, it would seem to be the opposite. I always loved the water, so naturally, when I was about eleven years old, I joined a swim team. I was not the most talented or athletic swimmer out there. But I was good enough to make my high school team and become captain my senior year. Why am I mentioning this? Because I remember that those years were when I had a healthy relationship with movement. Even in high school, when I was more acutely aware of dieting and the girls around me were calculating calories burned, I somehow managed to just truly love swimming and how it made my body feel. I loved being in the water, I loved how free it felt to move, and I loved the challenge of trying to move my body faster and faster. That is what joyful movement feels like for me.

As we all know, there are many benefits to movement. But people often feel discouraged when it comes to exercise and assume that they haven't found the right class or type of exercise when they don't see immediate physical transformation. If your body isn't changing fast enough, what's the point? But I offer a different approach: if you were to begin an exercise routine knowing in advance that no matter what you did, your body wouldn't change physically, then what movement would you choose? Would it still be jogging? Maybe it would be dancing, or even afternoon kickball. Exercise is beneficial, but movement without joy typically isn't sustainable. Not to mention that the hardest form of movement or the hardest class doesn't always translate to the best choice for you individually.

Joyful ideas to try out:

- Taking a stroll in the park

- Gardening

- Hiking

- Bike riding

- Taking a yoga class

- Strength training

- Dancing (even around your kitchen)

- Going for a run

- Joining a local sports team

- Taking a martial arts class

- Jump rope

- Roller skating

- Swimming

THE MYTH OF 10,000 STEPS

CliffsNotes: Ten thousand steps a day started as a marketing gimmick in 1965 Japan when a pedometer company released, in English, the 10,000-Step Meter, launched with the slogan "Let's walk 10,000 steps a day."[5] There was no rhyme or reason for the 10k except great marketing.

The concept took off, as many fitness trackers and smartphones have the goal of getting people to 10k steps. But lo and behold, it turns out people are different and not everyone can hit that number, and we also know now that the number is unnecessary. The idea is to be less sedentary, and we don't have to go to extreme lengths in order to do that. One study found that for women ages 62–101, walking approximately 4,400 steps a day was associated with a 41 percent reduction in mortality compared with walking 2,700 steps a day. Walking around 7,500 steps was associated with a 85 percent reduction.[6]

So, is 10k a day a bad thing? Absolutely not. In a separate study, with participants aged 40 and older, the conclusion was that a greater number of steps per day was significantly associated with lower all-cause mortality. I, too, love the challenge of walking more and getting in steps. I am also fortunate enough to live in the walkable city of New York, so I enjoy walking just to get outside. And I now treat walking as a joyful activity. I'm not disappointed with myself for not reaching a certain number and recognize when my body needs rest.

There are, of course, plenty of other options, and it depends on what you personally find joyful. Outdoor activities might seem more accessible, but it depends on the safety of your environment. Going to communal places of movement, such as gyms and fitness studios, is also an option, but access depends on one's finances. I will also mention that if someone doesn't have a socially accepted body, they might feel unwelcome in these environments and might choose to forgo exercise and movement altogether. Movement, like food, is a complicated topic, and depending on individual factors, it might not be as easy as "just take a few minutes a day," as we're encouraged. As always, do what's best for you. It might not look like what everyone else is doing.

Instead of thinking of exercise as a regimented activity and something you have to be dripping with sweat from in order to be beneficial, it would be helpful to find ways to move your body that you personally enjoy. The more you enjoy doing something, the more you will participate in that activity. What movement do you enjoy? What feels joyful to you?

_____

_____

_____

_____

_____

CHAPTER TEN

FINDING BODY ACCEPTANCE

In a society that profits from your self-doubt, liking yourself
is a rebellious act.
                    —Caroline Caldwell[1]

Having a body is hard. It requires so much work, and it is so
incredibly needy. It doesn't allow you to just take a day off. You
need to feed it. You need to hydrate it. You need to wash it. You
need to clothe it. You need to move it. You need to take it to different humans for inspections, maintenance, and checkups. You
need to let it rest. And there is no one-size-fits-all manual that
you receive at birth for guidance. You have to figure this shit out
on your own. To complicate things even more, there is so much
conflicting information that it's hard to know what is meant for
you as an individual.

Then there are layers of intersectionality to consider. It's incredibly hard to be a woman in this society. It's even harder to be
a Black woman. We can add more levels of intersectionality with
being part of the LGBTQ+ community, being disabled, having
a larger body, and more. Let me just say that it *shouldn't* be hard,
because society should accommodate diversity and diverse bodies with diverse needs, but we live in a white, hetero, cisgender,

nondisabled, thin, patriarchal society, which makes it difficult. Loving ourselves when we are put in the other box in society is hard. It makes sense to want to conform and assimilate.

I love unapologetically taking up space. Mostly because for so many years I tried to do the exact opposite. I felt uncomfortable in my first career, so trying to diminish and shrink myself made sense, though not at the time, of course. In a weird way I wish twenty-four-year-old Shana had the social media she does now. Instagram wasn't really the platform it is today, and Twitter was barely off and running (I'm *really* dating myself here). Social media has its problems, but it has also opened a whole other level of accessible learning and bonding over shared lived experiences. I had no idea that what I was experiencing at work were microaggressions and basic mean-girl bullying. I had no idea what an introvert was, or that I was one. Where I just thought I was shy around certain people, I now know I felt drained by them. I also now know that as a Black woman I was not allowed to be introverted. I was expected to perform and be entertaining to my colleagues, and when I wasn't, I was brushed aside. "When we aren't overly talkative, overly expressive, and living our lives out loud as they expect, I believe our lack of animation and conversation can be misread as [being] mean, unfriendly, angry, unhappy, and even unengaged. The trouble with this is that this misperception can impact leaderships' decisions about raises, bonuses, promotions, and key assignments,"[2] says Jeri Bingham, the founder and host of *Hush Loudly* and the creator of Black Introvert Week. That is incredibly on point. I remember my own experiences at work with constantly being labeled by my coworkers, who didn't even attempt to get to know me.

When I was working in fashion, a manager once told me,

"You're making some of the team uncomfortable. I honestly was so scared to even have this conversation with you on this because you make *me* nervous." Nervous laughter. "In what way, exactly?" I asked. Mind you, I'm not sure where I got the courage to ask this—because remember, I was still trying to shrink and not be seen (or heard)—but I did. The best part of that conversation was the pause when I asked that. You could hear a pin drop. She didn't know and couldn't really explain it, but she just *felt* uncomfortable. The icing on the cake was that this was a supervisor, and someone who's above you on a work ladder telling you that you make them nervous is, well, telling. This gave me all the information I needed on how I was being perceived. I wish I had seen the hundreds of other Black women who currently tweet and post about scenarios such as this one. I wish I knew I wasn't alone. But instead, I shut my mouth and shrank physically and mentally some more.

• BODY POSITIVITY ISN'T ENOUGH •

We can't all self-love our way out of the way society treats us. What I was going through at work couldn't be changed by repeating affirmations in the mirror to feel better. It couldn't be changed by telling myself it's okay to eat the foods I liked. It required a societal facelift and also a personal realization that the microaggressions were not a reflection of my worth as a human. I honestly don't remember the exact aha moment when I started gaining confidence and stopped shrinking physically and mentally. I was in my thirties, for sure, and it was around the time I switched careers and began having an actual passion for my new career. This didn't fix society, of course, but it gave me a new outlook on it. In my opinion, the body positivity movement is like the affirmations that we are told to say to ourselves in the mirror to fix everything. Don't get me wrong—affirmations and positive reinforcement are great, but we need more.

We have to be honest here: the mainstream body positivity movement does little to address the stigma that folks in larger bodies face. Many people only feel comfortable looking at and accepting certain types of bodies. There is always a "but," and you can often see this in social media debates. "I'm all for people being treated with respect, *but* they are unhealthy" is still stigmatizing. The phrase should be "I'm all for people being treated with respect," full stop. Period, end quote. The "but" just negates everything that was said in the first part of the sentence. Not to mention that bodies aren't business cards. We as a society treat them as such, but they shouldn't be. There never seems to be outrage for the actor who is harming their body with disordered habits for roles. There never seems to be outrage over athletes who are placing their bodies in harm's way for their sport. Whenever there is talk of eating disorders in society and how normalized disordered eating is, there is always the counter or straw man argument (an argument that avoids the opponent's actual argument and instead argues against an inaccurate caricature of it[3]) of "Well, what about obesity?" Aside from how problematic that statement is, continuing to view only one body type as a problem confirms the weight bias and stigma regarding how we view bodies in society.

I personally am not an ally for body positivity because it has become a movement for thin, white, able-bodied, cis women who have belly rolls when bending over. A few years ago, I found those images empowering, and I was all about #bodypositivity. I used to admire the creators who were adamant about "that lower belly is not actually fat, it's your uterus!" and "Love yourself! We all have a roll when we sit down." Oh yeah, this all made me feel so good, because as a thin, able-bodied, cis woman myself, I found it relatable. Then I started listening, learning, and reflecting. The more I began to dig deeper, the more I realized I was an outlier in this movement. And this is in no way meant to take away or discredit any particular influencer or creator, but body positivity has taken a serious detour from its original roots.

The more I began really looking into healthism and seeing how society places blame on the individual instead of the systems in place, the more I realize how simply learning to love every roll might not be possible. I have never lived in a larger body, nor do I pretend to understand what it is truly like to feel discrimination based on size. I want to make it clear that I am not speaking for a demographic when there are plenty of fat liberation creators (especially Black creators) who are more than qualified to speak on the problems of anti-fatness in society. I also understand that the demographic is not a monolith and not everyone shares the same viewpoint. There are some who feel better when pursuing weight loss, and that's their personal choice to make. My role as a health professional is to take my knowledge of nutrition and its effects on the body while also taking someone's lived experience into consideration when providing tools for their toolbox. It is not my place to judge someone for the choices they make, because simply put, I'm not in their body.

• BODY RESPECT •

I sometimes miss my twenty-four-year-old body. Yes, the one that I described as going through disordered eating and the toxic work environment. I sometimes miss her. I sometimes miss the way clothes fit. I sometimes miss the way I had control in some aspect of my life when I was micromanaging my food. I sometimes miss the compliments I received. It's messed up, but it's sometimes that toxic relationship that I miss. *Sometimes.*

When discussing healing our relationship with ourselves, whether that's with food or our body, we don't talk about the mourning period and how it never fully disappears. There was a piece of us that was happy when we were in that toxic relationship, for whatever reason. Life was easier somehow, and who wouldn't want that? Clothes fit better, or maybe you were treated better in society. This is normal and, in my opinion, not talked about enough, because social media makes the journey feel as though there is an endpoint, and unfortunately, that's not (usually) the case.

We live in a world where pushing ourselves to an extreme is normal and encouraged. It's hard to find body peace and acceptance when the world is constructed in a way that celebrates shrinking and contorting. I remember the state of my mental health during this period of endless contortion. I also remember my physical state with the weakness and the missed menstruation. When I first had my aha moment of healing and finding peace, it wasn't a feeling of loving every inch and acceptance of my physicality but a feeling of respect. It was as if I entered an internalized agreement with my body that I was going to respect it. I didn't promise to love it 24/7, but I did promise to show it respect. Respect to me means care, compassion, and nourishment.

There is a quote I often think about from an anonymous source I come across on the Internet from time to time:

Did you ever realize how much your body loves you? I mean, it's always trying to keep you alive. That's all your body has to live for. Your body is making sure you breathe while you sleep, stopping cuts from bleeding, fixing broken bones, finding ways to beat the illness that might get you. Your body literally loves you so much. It's time to start loving your body back.

—Anonymous[4]

Now, I get how this might sound nonsensical if you have a chronic illness or disease or some condition that makes you feel at constant war with your body. I say this on my social media posts, so I'll give the same disclaimer here: not everything is for everyone. There are more than eight billion people on this planet, so no, not everything is going to resonate with us, and that's more than okay. However, we all still need to take care of ourselves as best we can. I also understand that these basic necessities aren't so basic for everyone. It's hard to respect yourself with nourishment if you are struggling with food insecurity. It's hard to respect yourself with clothing when mass retailers often don't make clothes past a certain size. We can't self-love our way out of systemic oppression, but we can do our best and show compassion to ourselves.

Body neutrality goes hand-in-hand with body respect, as both recognize the futility of attempting to get to a place of loving every inch of ourselves all the time, because that's impossible for any of us; however, we can feel neutral about our bodies. We can still respect our bodies. I might be having a bad body image day and feel meh about myself, but I also acknowledge that I should take care of myself the best way I can. That is body respect. I can respect my body because I know it's working against all odds to keep me alive. I can respect my body because I know that even though I feel at war with it, it is doing so much for me.

So how does one get to a place of neutrality or respect? It sounds much more attainable than positivity but can still be difficult.

• SHOW YOURSELF COMPASSION •

Showing compassion to ourselves is a way we can connect with ourselves internally. It means having grace, forgiveness, and acceptance even when the situations are not optimal. It requires knowing our worth is unconditional even when we are handed undesirable circumstances. Psychologist Dr. Kristin Neff was one of the first researchers to measure and operationally define the term *self-compassion*. I find her definition to be spot-on: "Instead of mercilessly judging and criticizing yourself for various inadequacies or shortcomings, self-compassion means you are kind and understanding when confronted with personal failings—after all, who ever said you were supposed to be perfect?"[5]

I don't believe there's such a thing as perfection. I say quite often that there's no such thing as perfect eating whenever I'm asked a generalized question on nutrition, but I believe that applies to humans in every aspect. Yes, we can aspire to be the best versions of ourselves, but often we are chasing an idea of what we should and shouldn't be doing in order to look like an unrealistic aesthetic. And when we don't live up to that idea, we get discouraged and our self-esteem takes a hit. Perfection doesn't exist, and it's okay to offer yourself grace and compassion because you're human.

• BODIES CHANGE, SELF-WORTH DOES NOT •

You have not failed if your body has changed. In fact, change means that you're human. Our bodies can change due to many reasons, such as age, stress, trauma, medications, illnesses, and medical conditions. I am not in any way saying that change is easy or comfortable, but it happens. Since we are made to believe that we should look the same throughout our lives, when we change, we often feel as though we are not living up to a certain version of perfectionism.

Part of having body respect is not attaching our worth to our appearance. We often don't realize that we do this, but when we don't live up to the version of ourselves that we have in our heads, we think we failed, and we think ourselves less than. We think we did something wrong or that we're not prioritizing our health.

We're not supposed to look the same throughout our lives. I cringe at every article I come across that advertises how to get your twenty-year-old body back, as if aging was the worst possible thing to happen to humans. Even if our weight changed drastically, that doesn't translate into something negative. Not all weight gain is bad, and not all weight loss is good. Gaining weight can mean recovery from years of restriction; it can mean that your body is healing. It can mean that you are trusting your body and learning how to properly nourish it. It can mean that you are coming into peace and accepting your genetic makeup and size. None of that is negative, and no matter what lies we are told by society about expecting to maintain our physicality throughout life and the thin ideal, our worth as humans has nothing to do with our body.

• SHUT DOWN THE BODY TALK •

It's become a societal norm to talk about bodies like they are trending news topics. Every little change on a celebrity's body is dissected as if it's news. But you don't have to be in the public eye to know how common body checking (information received about and comparison of our physicality) is. Sometimes it's in the form of self-deprecation and we offer negative comments about ourselves before anyone else can say anything, but quite often we hear unsolicited comments from others.

The thing about receiving comments on your body is that even though it's normalized and even though some comments might be positive, they are still quite uncomfortable. I remember receiving an influx of commentary that was positive during my disordered eating days, but it was still somewhat humiliating because I realized that I was on display. We must realize that we don't know someone's struggles, and constantly talking about someone's body and the changes in that body means we might be forcing them to talk about something they're not ready to or want to disclose.

Shutting down triggering talk and enforcing boundaries can be especially hard when it comes to family, because we know that commentary, no matter how uncouth or out of pocket, is probably coming from a place of love and concern. This is also cultural, as there are many times family members will make a comment on our appearance as a greeting before even saying hello. "Wow, you've gotten big—enjoying all that good food, huh?" "So skinny! All bones. Let me feed you." Coming from a Caribbean culture that does this, let me say that just because that is normal doesn't make it okay. We don't have to encourage broken systems—we can try to change them.

So what are some counter exchanges to these comments that can shut them all down? Here are some suggestions:

1. **Straight to the point:** *My body isn't a topic of discussion.*

2. **Uncomfortable but wants to make feelings known politely:** Change the topic of conversation. *Did you all catch the Yankees game yesterday?*

3. **For the family concerned with health:** *Thanks, but I am taking care of my health the best way I can. I'm not discussing my body anymore.*

4. **You've made your boundaries known before and they are being ignored:** *Remember when I said before that I didn't want to talk about my body? That hasn't changed.*

5. **You're just over it all:** Ignore the commentary with silence. The message will be received if you're ignoring them.

Even with the variety of responses we can give to our family, establishing boundaries isn't easy. We don't want to hurt anyone's feelings even if ours were hurt, and we may also feel as though we aren't being respectful if we say something negative. This is when nuance and figuring out a way that works for you personally comes into play. Having community and family is important, of course, but so is having your mental health.

• SOCIAL MEDIA •

I have a love/hate relationship with social media. There is no doubt that it can be a place of learning, which is beneficial. Social media is where I learned about the grip that diet culture has on us and the pipeline of white supremacy that it stemmed from. It is also a place that can make me feel less than or not enough. We tend to compare ourselves with others, and that is compounded on social media. There are creators and influencers of every genre and category imaginable, but not all content is created equally. There is nothing wrong with health and wellness, of course, but there are different ways that health is presented to us. Social media, like society, promotes unrealistic beauty and body standards, and at the same time congratulates all our attempts—in actuality, disordered eating tactics—at trying to achieve them. There seems to be a "do as I do and you will look like me" vibe that is apparent in posts.

We are bombarded with not only information but also images that are all available at our fingertips. Whether we are cognizant of it or not, we have a tendency to compare ourselves to what we see, which affects our mental health. Teens and young adults who reduced their social media use by 50 percent for just a few weeks saw significant improvement in how they felt about both their weight and their overall appearance compared with peers who maintained consistent levels of social media use.[6]

It's not just teenagers who are impressionable. One interview of active social media users aged twenty-eight to seventy-three found that

- 60 percent of people using social media reported that it has impacted their self-esteem in a negative way;

- 50 percent reported social media having negative effects on their relationships; and

- 80 percent reported that is easier to be deceived by others through their sharing on social media.[7]

In other words, it's very hard to keep up with the Joneses, because the Joneses aren't always forthcoming about their actual lifestyle. I see this comparison and contrast all the time in what-I-eat-in-a-day posts. Social media isn't always honest, so there is no way to tell if someone is being truthful about what they are actually consuming. Not to mention that what and how someone else eats doesn't automatically translate into what we should be eating and trying. It's rough out there, and many of us feel triggered or tired by the constant consumption of information. Many of us—myself included—are actually in need of social media breaks, but how can we tell? Here are some things to think about:

1. How do you feel when you're scrolling? Are you constantly getting triggered by posts? Social media should be fun, even if you're seeking to learn something. Constantly getting upset or discouraged when viewing posts can be a sign that you need a break.

2. Do you find yourself comparing and contrasting physicality or lifestyles? For example, your friend is on their third international trip this year, and you haven't even thought about vacation yet. Or the influencer that you don't know personally just got engaged and you just broke up with your partner. These scenarios can cause us to think we're behind or not doing something correctly in life.

3. You're bored and have a habit of reaching for the phone. This is many of us, myself included. There are many times when I'm scrolling and just liking without actually reading and taking in what's in front of me. Yes,

it's possible to take breaks from a busy day by scrolling, but it's also best to realize when you are mindlessly consuming information.

4. Is your phone the first thing you reach for in the morning and the last thing you look at at night? If apps are taking up our free time, with the constant need to view our feed and post and display our lives, we should think about taking a break. Social media is not the same thing as building in-person social connections.

These are just some things to think about, because our mental health is extremely important. Breaks are most welcome, of course, but if you notice that you feel the same way viewing the same accounts constantly, I recommend also detoxing and decluttering your feed. This is the one and only detox I will ever recommend, FYI:

1. Unfollow accounts that trigger you. Notice how certain accounts make you feel. If you don't feel comfortable unfollowing, you can always mute.

2. Declutter and reorganize your feed by diversifying. Find accounts of topics that interest you but follow accounts you normally wouldn't. Intentionally seek out different bodies and demographics. Social media can be a great learning tool, but only if that learning is intentional. Sometimes we have to acknowledge those feelings and sit with discomfort. We are being given information that we are not used to seeing or don't quite understand fully. We are seeing bodies that aren't represented equally in the media.

3. Report accounts that are spreading harmful rhetoric such as extremely low calorie counting, meal skipping, and/or pro-ana (anorexia) content. Many social media platforms also allow you to flag content you're uninterested in so they don't keep showing and advertising it to you.

• YOU'RE HUMAN •

Our bodies aren't home improvement projects. We shouldn't look for quick solutions to problems. Our body is our forever home. Does our home require work? Yes. However, we aren't a piece of architecture, we are living and breathing forms. We are humans with ever-changing needs. An uncomfortable part of being human is that our bodies will change. Our bodies age, certain parts might stop functioning consistently, some bodies grow other humans inside them, some bodies change because the medications that we need change our physicality, and some bodies hold on to the trauma that we as humans face. We are constantly working to fix ourselves. What if we really stopped and thought about these societal ideals and how unrealistic and unnecessary they are?

I'm not here to tell you how to love yourself unconditionally, especially when living in a world that will tell you otherwise. I'm also saying this as a fellow human who is also living in this society and who also has bad days. To quote Megan Thee Stallion, "Bad bitches have bad days, too."[8] It's incredibly frustrating to live in a society that is hyperfocused on appearance, and people are entitled to the quick fixes that make them feel better about themselves. However, my hope is that we can all reach some level of peace with ourselves. Think about how much time and effort it takes to fight ourselves. We know that diets are fruitless, yet we embark on them anyway. We know the side effects of medications and surgeries, but they are recommended anyway. I understand how hard it is to live in this society that treats us based on what our body looks like. I understand how much easier it feels to try to assimilate rather than go against the norm. But this constant fight that we have with ourselves is not peace.

Peace is when we nourish our bodies with food that is accessible to us and that we enjoy. That nourishment is in the form of vitamins and minerals but also comfort and joy. It's a tie to our heritage and family traditions and takes the form of our social connections. Peace is moving your body in a way that feels good to you and that brings you actual joy. It's knowing that your body is unique and individual and there is no one-size-fits-all approach to how it's cared for. There is peace once we realize that there is no such thing as perfection, because perfection is a made-up concept in order for us to buy (literally) into the idea that we need to constantly work toward unrealistic goals with an ever-changing bull's-eye.

Food, nutrition, and the body are often viewed with a binary lens and a one-size-fits-all approach to health to strive for this idea of perfection that is advertised to us by society. To achieve it, we normalize disordered eating behaviors and lifestyle practices. What we need to remember is that nutrition is not about relying on black-and-white rules but about honoring our individual genetic blueprint while also welcoming the feeling of comfort and joy with food. My hope is for everyone to realize that healthy eating is not restrictive eating. Healthy eating is not moralizing food when every single one of us needs to eat every day in order to survive. There is not a right or wrong approach—but please always season your food.

We are all humans trying to survive in a world that is constantly challenging us with hurdles to leap over. Some of us have more hurdles due to different circumstances, but the most we can do is try to take care of ourselves as best we can. That care and compassion will look different to all of us. All I want to say is that you're doing okay. You're human.

ACKNOWLEDGMENTS

I remember receiving the email asking if I was interested in writing a book. Me, write a whole book? I posted and talked about whatever I was feeling and thinking on social media. That imposter syndrome slowly creeping in, of thinking there were so many dietitians already writing with much more experience than me. However, I still knew that I had a voice and a way of using words that resonated with people. So with that, I want to thank my editor, Ronnie, for that initial email nudge of "You should write," and for somehow turning it into the book that it is today. Thank you to my agent, Laura Lee, for your guidance and support. The dream literary team.

The non-diet and weight-inclusive space and community has been amazing and supportive. Thank you so much for the acceptance and the constant and ever-evolving learning. To the social justice, fat, and marginalized identity leaders and activists, a huge shout-out and thank-you for your wisdom and teachings on these subjects. Being in these spaces is an uphill battle because it's fighting against "the norm." But we're here and standing strong. It's amazing to find community with like-minded individuals who are fighting for the same cause. I'm thankful for the forums, events, and RD group chats.

Thank you so much to Flory, Iliana, Jessica (Tara), Catherine, Lorraine, Eling, Lara, Barbara, Sharon, Chrissy, and Stephanie.

You all have been amazing friends with the constant encouraging check-ins, late-night texts and laughs, and dinner distraction talks. I met you all through different parts of my life, and I couldn't ask for a more caring and loving friend circle. You all rock!

Mom, Dad, I wrote a book! Your only daughter wrote a book, and I couldn't have done it without either of you. Mom, you were always encouraging me to do more and find something I love. I hate to admit that you were right. Dad, I can't wait to read this to you. I hope this makes up for all the early-morning drives to swim practice. Love you both so much.

Thank you so much to the online community for the ongoing support. I write what I think and feel, and that seems to resonate with a few of you. You have allowed me to create a community, but you all are the ones who fill it and interact with it regularly. I feel grateful for your continued support.

NOTES

Introduction

1. *Merriam-Webster*, s.v. "culture (n.)," accessed September 3, 2023, https://www.merriam-webster.com/dictionary/culture.

2. Sarah Budhiwianto et al., "Global Prevalence of Eating Disorders in Nutrition and Dietetic University Students: A Systematic Scoping Review," *Nutrients* 15, no. 10 (2023): 2317, https://doi.org/10.3390/nu15102317.

3. K. Hinterland et al., Community Health Profiles 2018, "Brooklyn Community District 17: East Flatbush" (New York: 2018), 1–20, https://www.nyc.gov/assets/doh/downloads/pdf/data/2018chp-bk17.pdf.

4. K. Hinterland et al., Community Health Profiles 2018, "Brooklyn Community District 6: Park Slope and Carroll Gardens" (New York: 2018), 1–20, https://www.nyc.gov/assets/doh/downloads/pdf/data/2018chp-bk6.pdf.

5. Robert Crawford, "Healthism and the Medicalization of Everyday Life," *International Journal of Social Determinants of Health and Health Services* 10, no. 3 (July 1980): 365–88, https://doi.org/10.2190/3h2h-3xjn-3kay-g9ny.

Chapter One: Why Diets Don't Work

1. EricT_CulinaryLore, "What Is the Origin of the Word Diet?" Culinary Lore, August 26, 2014, https://culinarylore.com/food-history:origin-of-the-word-diet/.

2. *Merriam-Webster*, s.v. "diet (*n.*) (1)," accessed August 27, 2022, https://www.merriam-webster.com/dictionary/diet#h1.

3. Bryan Stierman et al., "Special Diets among Adults: United States, 2015–2018," *NCHS Data Brief* 389 (November 2020).

4. Rena R. Wing and Suzanne Phelan, "Long-Term Weight Loss Maintenance," *American Journal of Clinical Nutrition* 82, no. 1 (July 1, 2005): 222S–25S, https://doi.org/10.1093/ajcn/82.1.222s; D. D. Hensrud et al., "A Prospective Study of Weight Maintenance in Obese Subjects Reduced to Normal Body Weight without Weight-Loss Training," *American Journal of Clinical Nutrition* 60, no. 5 (November 1994): 688–94, https://doi.org/10.1093/ajcn/60.5.688; and Zata M. Vickers et al., "Medicare's Search for Effective Obesity Treatments: Diets Are Not the Answer," *American Psychologist* 62, no. 3 (April 1, 2007): 220–33, https://doi.org/10.1037/0003-066x.62.3.220.

5. Rebecca Stamp, "Average Person Will Try 126 Fad Diets in Their Lifetime, Poll Claims," *Independent*, January 8, 2020, https://www.independent.co.uk/life-style/diet-weight-loss-food-unhealthy-eating-habits-a9274676.html.

6. A. Janet Tomiyama, Britt Ahlstrom, and Traci Mann, "Long-Term Effects of Dieting: Is Weight Loss Related to Health?" *Social and Personality Psychology Compass* 7, no. 12 (December 2013): 861–77, https://doi.org/10.1111/spc3.12076.

7. Milan Obradovic et al., "Leptin and Obesity: Role and Clinical Implication," *Frontiers in Endocrinology* 12 (May 2021), https://doi.org/10.3389/fendo.2021.585887.

8. Leah M. Kalm and Richard D. Semba, "They Starved So That Others Be Better Fed: Remembering Ancel Keys and the Minnesota Experiment," *Journal of Nutrition* 135, no. 6 (June 2005): 1347–52, https://doi.org/10.1093/jn/135.6.1347.

9. David B. Baker and Natacha Keramidas, "The Psychology of Hunger," *Monitor on Psychology* 44, no. 9 (October 2013): 66, https://www.apa .org/monitor/2013/10/hunger.

10. Agnese Mariotti, "The Effects of Chronic Stress on Health: New Insights into the Molecular Mechanisms of Brain–Body Communication," *Future Science OA* 1, no. 3 (June 2015), https://doi.org/10.4155 /fso.15.21.

11. "Weight Cycling Is Associated with a Higher Risk of Death," Endocrine Society, November 29, 2018, https://www.endocrine.org /news-and-advocacy/news-room/2018/weight-cycling-is-associated -with-a-higher-risk-of-death.

12. Richard L. Atkinson et al., "Weight Cycling," *Journal of the American Medical Association* 272, no. 15 (October 1994): 1196–202, https:// jamanetwork.com/journals/jama/article-abstract/380893.

13. "What Are Eating Disorders?" National Eating Disorders Association, accessed January 18, 2023, https://www.nationaleatingdisorders.org /what-are-eating-disorders.

14. "What Is Disordered Eating?" Academy of Nutrition and Dietetics, February 28, 2020, https://www.eatright.org/health/diseases-and-con ditions/eating-disorders/what-is-disordered-eating.

15. *Diagnostic and Statistical Manual of Mental Disorders*, 5th Edition, ebook (American Psychiatric Association, 2013).

16. Jonathan R. Scarff, "Orthorexia Nervosa: An Obsession with Healthy Eating," *Federal Practitioner* 34, no. 6 (June 2017): 36–39, https:// pubmed.ncbi.nlm.nih.gov/30766283.

17. Johanna Sander, Markus Moessner, and Stephanie Bauer, "Depression, Anxiety, and Eating Disorder–Related Impairment: Moderators in Female Adolescents and Young Adults," *International Journal of Environmental Research and Public Health* 18, no. 5 (March 2021): 2779, https://doi.org/10.3390/ijerph18052779.

18. Lauren Edmonds, "Channing Tatum Says He Almost Didn't Film *Magic Mike 3* Because 'You Have to Starve Yourself,'" *Business Insider*, February 19, 2022, https://www.insider.com

/channing-tatum-you-have-to-starve-yourself-magic-mike
-body-2022-2#:~:text=look%20like%20that.-,Even%20if%20
you%20do%20work%20out%2C%20to%20be%20that%20
kind,lean%2C%20it's%20actually%20healthy.%22.

19. Simrin Sangha et al., "Eating Disorders in Males: How Primary Care Providers Can Improve Recognition, Diagnosis, and Treatment," *American Journal of Men's Health* 13, no. 3 (June 2019), https://doi .org/10.1177/1557988319857424.

20. Olivia J. Williams, "Sustenance Abuse: Anorexia, Bulimia, and Black Women," Washington University Open Scholarship, n.d., https:// openscholarship.wustl.edu/mcleod/8.

21. "What Is an Eating Disorder: Types, Symptoms, Risks, and Causes," Eating Disorder Hope, March 25, 2023, https://www.eatingdisorder hope.com/information/eating-disorder.

22. Katherine L. Morgan-Lowes et al., "The Relationships between Perfectionism, Anxiety, and Depression across Time in Paediatric Eating Disorders," *Eating Behaviors* 34 (August 2019): 101305, https://doi .org/10.1016/j.eatbeh.2019.101305.

Chapter Two: The Hamster Wheel of Diet Culture

1. Research and Markets, "Overview of the $58 Billion US Weight Loss Market 2022," *GlobeNewswire*, March 23, 2022, https://www. globenewswire.com/en/news-release/2022/03/23/2408315/28124/en /Overview-of-the-58-Billion-U-S-Weight-Loss-Market-2022.html.

2. "WW International, Inc., Announces Fourth Quarter and Full Year 2022 Results," Weight Watchers, March 6, 2023, https://corporate. ww.com/news-room/press-releases/news-details/2023/WW-Interna tional-Inc.-Announces-Fourth-Quarter-and-Full-Year-2022-Results /default.aspx.

3. Emily Cronkleton, "What Is Cellulite and How Can You Treat It?" Healthline, June 15, 2018, https://www.healthline.com/health/cellu lite.

4. William Barnhill, "The Cellulite Myth," *Washington Post*, March 6, 1985, https://www.washingtonpost.com/archive/lifestyle /wellness/1985/03/06/the-cellulite-myth/661b5726-da95-43ec -9459-dfabb505bbcf/.

5. Kelsey Miller, "Cellulite Isn't Real. This Is How It Was Invented," Refinery29, May 14, 2018, https://www.refinery29.com/en-us /what-is-cellulite-definition-fat-shaming-history.

6. Michael W. Sjoding et al., "Racial Bias in Pulse Oximetry Measurement," *New England Journal of Medicine* 383, no. 25 (December 2020): 2477–78, https://doi.org/10.1056/nejmc2029240.

7. Susan E. Short and Stefanie Mollborn, "Social Determinants and Health Behaviors: Conceptual Frames and Empirical Advances," *Current Opinion in Psychology* 5 (October 2015): 78–84, https://doi .org/10.1016/j.copsyc.2015.05.002.

8. Kevin D. Hall et al., "Energy Balance and Its Components: Implications for Body Weight Regulation," *American Journal of Clinical Nutrition* 95, no. 4 (April 2012): 989–94, https://doi.org/10.3945 /ajcn.112.036350.

9. Jessica Martino, Jennifer Pegg, and Elizabeth Pegg Frates, "The Connection Prescription: Using the Power of Social Interactions and the Deep Desire for Connectedness to Empower Health and Wellness," *American Journal of Lifestyle Medicine* 11, no. 6 (2017): 466–75, https://doi.org/10.1177/1559827615608788.

10. "Social Determinants of Health at CDC," Centers for Disease Control and Prevention, December 8, 2022, https://www.cdc.gov/about/sdoh /index.html.

11. Ibid.

12. "Racism and Health," Centers for Disease Control and Prevention, September 18, 2023, https://www.cdc.gov/minorityhealth/racism -disparities/index.html.

Chapter Three: We Cannot Be Carbon Copies of Each Other

1. Karen Asp, "50 Body Positivity Quotes, Because It Isn't Always Easy to Love Your Body 24/7," *Parade*, November 4, 2023, https://parade .com/1068565/karen-asp/body-positive-quotes/.

2. Online Etymology Dictionary, s.v. "obesity (n.)," accessed April 11, 2023, https://www.etymonline.com/word/obesity.

3. "Benefits of Physical Activity," Centers for Disease Control and Prevention, August 1, 2023, https://www.cdc.gov/physicalactivity/basics /pa-health/index.htm.

4. "Factors Affecting Weight & Health," National Institute of Diabetes and Digestive and Kidney Diseases, US Department of Health and Human Services, May 2023, https://www.niddk.nih.gov/health-infor mation/weight-management/adult-overweight-obesity/factors-affect ing-weight-health.

5. Laura Capon, "16 Ways Jennifer Lopez Makes 51 Look 31," *Cosmopolitan*, November 23, 2020, https://www.cosmopolitan.com/uk/beauty -hair/celebrity-hair-makeup/g10385940/jennifer-lopez-age/.

6. W Staff, "Jennifer Lopez's Rules for Ageless Beauty," *W*, July 24, 2019, https://www.wmagazine.com/beauty/jennifer-lopez-health-beauty -secrets.

7. Jasmine Fardouly and Lenny R. Vartanian, "Negative Comparisons about One's Appearance Mediate the Relationship between Facebook Usage and Body Image Concerns," *Body Image* 12 (January 2015): 82–88, https://doi.org/10.1016/j.bodyim.2014.10.004.

8. William F. Ferris and Nigel J. Crowther, "Once Fat Was Fat and That Was That: Our Changing Perspectives on Adipose Tissue," *Cardiovascular Journal of Africa* 22, no. 3 (May/June 2011): 147–54, https://doi .org/10.5830/cvja-2010-083.

9. Anne Hollander, "When Fat Was in Fashion," *New York Times*, October 23, 1977, https://www.nytimes.com/1977/10/23/archives/when -fat-was-in-fashion-abundant-flesh-was-a-thing-of-beauty-to.html.

10. Frank Q. Nuttall, "Body Mass Index: Obesity, BMI, and Health: A

Critical Review," *Nutrition Today* 50, no. 3 (May/June 2015): 117–28, https://doi.org/10.1097/nt.0000000000000092.

11. Lambert Adolphe Jacques Quetelet, *A Treatise on Man and the Development of His Faculties*, ebook (New York: Cambridge University Press, 2013), https://doi.org/10.1017/cbo9781139864909.

12. Donna Tafreshi, "Adolphe Quetelet and the Legacy of the 'Average Man' in Psychology," *History of Psychology* 25, no. 1 (February 2022): 34–55, https://doi.org/10.1037/hop0000202.

13. "About Adult BMI," Centers for Disease Control and Prevention, June 3, 2022, https://www.cdc.gov/healthyweight/assessing/bmi/adult_bmi/index.html.

14. A. Janet Tomiyama et al., "How and Why Weight Stigma Drives the Obesity 'Epidemic' and Harms Health," *BMC Medicine* 16, no. 1 (August 2018), https://doi.org/10.1186/s12916-018-1116-5.

15. Susan B. Racette, Susan S. Deusinger, and Robert H. Deusinger, "Obesity: Overview of Prevalence, Etiology, and Treatment," *Physical Therapy & Rehabilitation Journal* 83, no. 3 (March 2003): 276–88, https://doi.org/10.1093/ptj/83.3.276.

16. "Denial of Insurance," Council on Size and Weight Discrimination, http://cswd.org/denial-of-insurance.

17. Elizabeth Cohen and Anne McDermott, "Who's Fat? New Definition Adopted," CNN, June 17, 1998, http://www.cnn.com/HEALTH/9806/17/weight.guidelines/.

18. "What Is Atypical Anorexia Nervosa: Symptoms, Causes, and Treatment," Eating Disorder Hope, August 30, 2021, https://www.eatingdisorderhope.com/information/atypical-anorexia.

19. Susan M. Sawyer et al., "Physical and Psychological Morbidity in Adolescents with Atypical Anorexia Nervosa," *Pediatrics* 137, no. 4 (April 2016): e20154080, https://doi.org/10.1542/peds.2015-4080.

20. Tomiyama et al., "How and Why Weight Stigma Drives the Obesity 'Epidemic.'"

21. Christopher H. Warner et al., "Military Family Physician Attitudes

toward Treating Obesity," *Military Medicine* 173, no. 10 (October 2008): 978–84, https://doi.org/10.7205/milmed.173.10.978.

22. Rebecca M. Puhl and Chelsea A. Heuer, "Obesity Stigma: Important Considerations for Public Health," *American Journal of Public Health* 100, no. 6 (June 2010): 1019–28, https://doi.org/10.2105/ajph.2009.159491.

23. Tomiyama et al., "How and Why Weight Stigma Drives the Obesity 'Epidemic.'"

24. Puhl and Heuer, "Obesity Stigma."

25. Hilary George-Parkin, "Size, by the Numbers," *Racked*, June 5, 2018, https://www.racked.com/2018/6/5/17380662/size-numbers-average-woman-plus-market.

26. Gianluca Russo, "Why Don't 'Size-Inclusive' Brands Carry Plus Sizes in Stores?" *Refinery29*, July 12, 2022, https://www.refinery29.com/en-us/2022/03/10874398/plus-size-in-store-shopping-brands.

27. "Universal Declaration of Human Rights," United Nations, n.d., https://www.un.org/en/about-us/universal-declaration-of-human-rights.

28. "Mom Shares Disappointing Experience at Universal Studios Due to Lack of Size-Inclusive Rides," Yahoo! Life, n.d., https://www.yahoo.com/lifestyle/mom-shares-disappointing-experience-universal-211039066.html.

29. Anna Kaplan, "Why Passengers Are Fighting over Airline Seat Size Ahead of the Holidays," Today.com, November 3, 2022, https://www.today.com/news/faa-airplane-seat-size-rcna55410.

30. "Body Measurements," Centers for Disease Control and Prevention, September 10, 2021, https://www.cdc.gov/nchs/fastats/body-measurements.htm.

31. Aubrey Gordon, "Fat People Usually Have to Buy a Second Plane Seat. That Has to Change," *BuzzFeed News*, January 17, 2023, https://www.buzzfeednews.com/article/aubreygordon/flying-while-fat.

32. Meridith Griffin, K. Alysse Bailey, and Kimberly J. Lopez,

"#BodyPositive? A Critical Exploration of the Body Positive Movement within Physical Cultures Taking an Intersectionality Approach," *Frontiers in Sports and Active Living* 4 (October 2022), https://doi.org/10.3389/fspor.2022.908580.

33. "About Us," National Association to Advance Fat Acceptance, n.d. https://naafa.org/about-us.

34. Gene Demby, "The Mothers Who Fought to Radically Reimagine Welfare," NPR, June 9, 2019, https://www.npr.org/sections/codeswitch/2019/06/09/730684320/the-mothers-who-fought-to-radically-reimagine-welfare.

35. Stephanie Yeboah, *Fattily Ever After: A Black Fat Girl's Guide to Living Life Unapologetically* (Berkeley, CA: Hardie Grant Publishing, 2020).

36. Da'Shaun L. Harrison, *Belly of the Beast: The Politics of Anti-Fatness as Anti-Blackness* (Berkeley, CA: North Atlantic Books, 2021).

37. Sonya Renee Taylor, *The Body Is Not an Apology: The Power of Radical Self-Love* (Oakland, CA: Berrett-Koehler Publishers, 2018).

38. Roxane Gay, *Hunger: A Memoir of (My) Body* (London: Hachette UK, 2017).

39. Aubrey Gordon, *What We Don't Talk About When We Talk About Fat* (Boston: Beacon Press, 2020).

40. Sabrina Strings, *Fearing the Black Body: The Racial Origins of Fat Phobia* (New York: NYU Press, 2019).

Chapter Four: Elitism of Health and Wellness

1. Melanie Whyte, "Self-Care Is Only the First Step to Wellness, Says Author Fariha Róisín in *Who Is Wellness For?*" POPSUGAR, October 14, 2022, https://www.popsugar.com/fitness/who-is-wellness-for-interview-with-author-fariha-roisin-48885446.

2. "NWI's Six Dimensions of Wellness," National Wellness Institute, accessed February 17, 2023, https://nationalwellness.org/resources/six-dimensions-of-wellness/.

3. "Constitution," World Health Organization, n.d., https://www.who .int/about/accountability/governance/constitution.

4. "In Goop Health," Goop, accessed May 7, 2023, https://goop.com /ingoophealth/.

5. Shaun Callaghan et al., "Feeling Good: The Future of the $1.5 Trillion Wellness Market," McKinsey & Company, April 8, 2021, https:// www.mckinsey.com/industries/consumer-packaged-goods/our-in sights/feeling-good-the-future-of-the-1-5-trillion-wellness-market.

6. "IFIC Survey: From 'Chemical-Sounding' to 'Clean': Consumer Perspectives on Food Ingredients," Food Insight, June 17, 2021, https:// foodinsight.org/ific-survey-from-chemical-sounding-to-clean-con sumer-perspectives-on-food-ingredients/.

7. "Statistics About Diabetes," American Diabetes Association, n.d., https://www.diabetes.org/about-us/statistics/about-diabetes.

8. Mary Smith, "Native Americans: A Crisis in Health Equity," American Bar Association, n.d., https://www.americanbar.org/groups/crsj /publications/human_rights_magazine_home/the-state-of-healthcare -in-the-united-states/native-american-crisis-in-health-equity/.

9. Meira Gebel, "Misinformation vs. Disinformation: What to Know about Each Form of False Information, and How to Spot Them Online," *Business Insider*, January 15, 2021, https://www.businessinsider .com/guides/tech/misinformation-vs-disinformation.

10. "Thanks a Billion!" TikTok, September 27, 2021, https://newsroom .tiktok.com/en-us/1-billion-people-on-tiktok.

11. Miles McEvoy, "Organic 101: What the USDA Organic Label Means," US Department of Agriculture, March 22, 2012, https://www .usda.gov/media/blog/2012/03/22/organic-101-what-usda-organic -label-means.

12. David Zaruk, "Risk, Hazard, and the Precautionary Principle: Why Europe Gets Crop Biotechnology and Chemical Regulation So Wrong," Genetic Literacy Project, July 24, 2018, https://geneticliteracyproject .org/2021/10/15/risk-hazard-and-precautionary-principle-why-eu rope-gets-crop-biotechnology-and-chemical-regulation-so-wrong.

13. FoodScienceBabe, "Hazard vs. Risk," Instagram, June 1, 2019, accessed August 10, 2022, https://www.instagram.com/p/ByLw62nAAbx/.

14. "2021 Food & Health Survey," Food Insight, May 19, 2021, https://foodinsight.org/2021-food-health-survey/.

15. Carlos Augusto Monteiro et al., "The UN Decade of Nutrition, the NOVA Food Classification, and the Trouble with Ultra-Processing," *Public Health Nutrition* 21, special issue 1 (March 2017): 5–17, https://doi.org/10.1017/s1368980017000234.

16. Mark Messina et al., "Perspective: Soy-Based Meat and Dairy Alternatives, Despite Classification as Ultra-Processed Foods, Deliver High-Quality Nutrition on Par with Unprocessed or Minimally Processed Animal-Based Counterparts," *Advances in Nutrition* 13, no. 3 (May 2022): 726–38, https://doi.org/10.1093/advances/nmac026.

17. Mandy Ferreira and Natalie Butler, "Are Fortified and Enriched Foods Healthy?" UNICEF Global Development Commons, November 26, 2019, https://unicef.org/resource/are-fortified-and-enriched-foods-healthy.

18. Jessica Caporuscio, PharmD, "What Are Food Deserts, and How Do They Impact Health?" MedicalNewsToday, June 22, 2020, https://www.medicalnewstoday.com/articles/what-are-food-deserts.

19. "Disability Impacts All of Us," Centers for Disease Control and Prevention, May 15, 2023, https://www.cdc.gov/ncbddd/disabilityandhealth/infographic-disability-impacts-all.html.

20. Marisa Sanfilippo, "What After-Hours Emails Really Do to Your Employees," *Business News Daily*, October 24, 2023, https://www.businessnewsdaily.com/9241-check-email-after-work.html.

21. Tyler Schmall, "Almost Half of Americans Consider Themselves 'Workaholics,'" *New York Post*, February 1, 2019, https://nypost.com/2019/02/01/almost-half-of-americans-consider-themselves-workaholics.

22. "10 Statistics on Work-Life Balance That May Surprise You," Apollo Technical, January 3, 2023, https://www.apollotechnical.com/statistics-on-work-life-balance/.

Chapter Five: Food Freedom Beyond "Just Eat the Cookie"

1. Ta-Nehisi Coates, *Between the World and Me* (London: One World, 2015).

2. "Bodily Autonomy: A Fundamental Right," United Nations Population Fund, March 16, 2022, https://www.unfpa.org/press/bodily-autonomy-fundamental-right.

3. "About the Association for Size Diversity and Health (ASDAH)," Association for Size Diversity and Health, accessed March 9, 2023, https://asdah.org/about-asdah/.

4. S. Guillaume et al., "Associations between Adverse Childhood Experiences and Clinical Characteristics of Eating Disorders," *Scientific Reports* 6 (2016): 35761, https://doi.org/10.1038/srep35761.

5. "Moya Bailey, *Misogynoir Transformed: Black Women's Digital Resistance*," Center for the Study of Race and Ethnicity in America, Brown University, n.d., https://www.brown.edu/academics/race-ethnicity/events/moya-bailey-%E2%80%9Cmisogynoir-transformed-black-women%E2%80%99s-digital-resistance%E2%80%9D.

6. Marcie Ward, RN, and Patti L. Ellis, RN, CPHRM, "Pediatrics: Addressing Social Determinants of Health and Adverse Childhood Experiences," The Doctors Company, accessed February 23, 2022, https://www.thedoctors.com/articles/pediatrics-addressing-social-determinants-of-health-and-adverse-childhood-experiences/.

7. D. W. Rowlands, Manann Donoghoe, and Andre M. Perry, "What the Lack of Premium Grocery Stores Says about Disinvestment in Black Neighborhoods," Brookings, April 11, 2023, https://www.brookings.edu/research/what-the-lack-of-premium-grocery-stores-says-about-disinvestment-in-black-neighborhoods.

8. "East Flatbush, Farragut & Rugby PUMA, NY," Data USA, n.d., https://datausa.io/profile/geo/east-flatbush-farragut-rugby-puma-ny.

9. K. Hinterland et al., Community Health Profiles 2018, "Brooklyn Community District 17: East Flatbush" (New York: 2018), 1–20, https://www.nyc.gov/assets/doh/downloads/pdf/data/2018chp-bk17.pdf.

10. Kevin B. O'Reilly, "AMA: Racism Is a Threat to Public Health," American Medical Association, November 16, 2020, https://www.ama-assn.org/delivering-care/health-equity/ama-racism-threat-public-health.

11. "Racial Equity," American Public Health Association, n.d., https://www.apha.org/topics-and-issues/health-equity/racism-and-health.

12. "What Is Epigenetics?" Centers for Disease Control and Prevention, August 15, 2022, https://www.cdc.gov/genomics/disease/epigenetics.htm.

13. Jenny Guidi et al., "Allostatic Load and Its Impact on Health: A Systematic Review," *Psychotherapy and Psychosomatics* 90, no. 1 (December 2020): 11–27, https://doi.org/10.1159/000510696.

Chapter Six: Intuitive Eating

1. Evelyn Tribole, "It's Common to Feel Conflicted upon Realizing You Are Full," EvelynTribole.com, April 8, 2019, https://www.evelyntribole.com/its-common-to-feel-conflicted-upon-realizing-you-are-full/.

2. "Demographics," Commission on Dietetic Registration, n.d., https://www.cdrnet.org/academy-commission-on-dietetic-registration-demographics.

3. David B. Baker and Natacha Keramidas, "The Psychology of Hunger," *Monitor on Psychology* 44, no. 9 (October 2013): 66, https://www.apa.org/monitor/2013/10/hunger.

4. Evelyn Tribole, "Definition of Intuitive Eating," IntuitiveEating.org, July 17, 2019, https://www.intuitiveeating.org/definition-of-intuitive-eating/.

5. Judy Klemesrud, "Don't Call It a Fat Camp," *New York Times*, August 4, 1975, https://www.nytimes.com/1975/08/04/archives/dont-call-it-a-fat-camp.html.

6. Susie Orbach, "Forty Years since *Fat Is a Feminist Issue*," *Guardian*, June 24, 2018, https://www.theguardian.com/society/2018/jun/24/forty-years-since-fat-is-a-feminist-issue.

7. Catherine Conroy, "Susie Orbach: 40 Years on, Fat Is Still a Feminist Issue," *Irish Times*, July 24, 2015, https://www.irishtimes.com /life-and-style/people/susie-orbach-40-years-on-fat-is-still-a-feminist -issue-1.2291162.

8. Frédérique R. E. Smink, Daphne van Hoeken, and Hans W. Hoek, "Epidemiology of Eating Disorders: Incidence, Prevalence, and Mortality Rates," *Current Psychiatry Reports* 14, no. 5 (May 2012): 406–14, https://doi.org/10.1007/s11920-012-0282-y.

9. "This Messy Magnificent Life: A Field Guide to Mind, Body, and Soul," GeneenRoth.com, n.d., https://geneenroth.com/books/.

10. Evelyn Tribole, MS, RDN, CEDRD-S, and Elyse Resch, MS, RDN, CEDRD-S, FAND, *Intuitive Eating: A Revolutionary Anti-Diet Approach*, 4th edition (New York: St. Martin's Essentials, 2020).

Chapter Seven: Find Your Own Path

1. Damian Barr, "'We Are Not All in the Same Boat. We Are All in the Same Storm. Some Are on Superyachts. Some Have Just the One Oar.'" DamianBarr.com, May 30, 2020, https://www.damianbarr .com/latest/https/we-are-not-all-in-the-same-boat.

2. Wang ZiMian et al., "Specific Metabolic Rates of Major Organs and Tissues across Adulthood: Evaluation by Mechanistic Model of Resting Energy Expenditure," *American Journal of Clinical Nutrition* 92, no. 6 (December 2010): 1,369–77, https://doi.org/10.3945 /ajcn.2010.29885.

3. Vanessa Caceres, "Weight Loss and Weight Gain Factors," *US News & World Report*, September 22, 2023, https://health.usnews.com/wellness /food/articles/factors-that-contribute-to-weight-loss-and-weight-gain.

4. Marc Sim et al., "Iron Considerations for the Athlete: A Narrative Review," *European Journal of Applied Physiology* 119 (May 2019): 1463–78, https://doi.org/10.1007/s00421-019-04157-y.

5. Steven H. Zeisel and Kerry-Ann da Costa, "Choline: An Essential Nutrient for Public Health," *Nutrition Reviews* 67, no. 11

(November 1, 2009): 615–23, https://doi.org/10.1111/j.1753 -4887.2009.00246.x.

6. Mark L. Heiman and Frank L. Greenway, "A Healthy Gastrointestinal Microbiome Is Dependent on Dietary Diversity," *Molecular Metabolism* 5, no. 5 (May 2016): 317–20, https://doi.org/10.1016/j.mol met.2016.02.005.

7. Philipp Mergenthaler et al., "Sugar for the Brain: The Role of Glucose in Physiological and Pathological Brain Function," *Trends in Neurosciences* 36, no. 10 (October 2013): 587–97, https://doi.org/10.1016/j .tins.2013.07.001.

8. "Benefits of Physical Activity," Centers for Disease Control and Prevention, August 1, 2023, https://www.cdc.gov/physicalactivity/basics /pa-health/index.htm.

9. *Legally Blonde*, directed by Robert Luketic (United States: Metro-Goldwyn-Mayer Distributing Corporation, 2001).

10. "SNAP Benefits," NYC Human Resources Administration," n.d., https://www.nyc.gov/site/hra/help/snap-benefits-food-program.page.

Chapter Eight: Reframe Your Approach to Food

1. Mel Schwartz, LCSW, "Our Words Matter," *Psychology Today*, April 10, 2019, https://www.psychologytoday.com/us/blog/shift -mind/201904/our-words-matter.

2. Jeremy Shapiro, PhD, "Finding Goldilocks: A Solution for Black-and-White Thinking," *Psychology Today*, May 1, 2020, https:// www.psychologytoday.com/us/blog/thinking-in-black-white-and -gray/202005/finding-goldilocks-solution-black-and-white-thinking.

3. *Merriam-Webster*, s.v. "cheat," accessed March 10, 2023, https://www .merriam-webster.com/dictionary/cheat.

4. *Merriam-Webster*, s.v. "good," accessed March 10, 2023, https://www .merriam-webster.com/dictionary/good.

5. Calodagh McCumiskey, "Words Can Affect Your Brain Functions,"

Irish Independent, June 12, 2020, https://www.independent.ie/regionals /corkman/lifestyle/words-can-affect-your-brain-functions-39280807 .html.

6. Peter Grinspoon, MD, "How to Recognize and Tame Your Cognitive Distortions," Harvard Health Publishing, May 4, 2022, https://www .health.harvard.edu/blog/how-to-recognize-and-tame-your-cognitive -distortions-202205042738.

7. "Dopamine," *Psychology Today,* n.d., https://www.psychologytoday .com/us/basics/dopamine.

Chapter Nine: Tools for Your Toolbox

1. "Thomas A. Edison Quotes," GoodReads, n.d., https://www.go odreads.com/quotes/8287-i-have-not-failed-i-ve-just-found-10-000 -ways-that.

2. Danielle Pacheco and Dr. Abhinav Singh, "Why Do We Need Sleep?" Sleep Foundation, December 8, 2023, https://www.sleepfoundation .org/how-sleep-works/why-do-we-need-sleep.

3. Maanvi Singh, "How Snobbery Helped Take the Spice Out of European Cooking," NPR, March 26, 2015, https://www.npr.org/sections /thesalt/2015/03/26/394339284/how-snobbery-helped-take-the -spice-out-of-european-cooking.

4. A. Susana Ramírez, PhD, MPH, et al., "Questioning the Dietary Acculturation Paradox: A Mixed-Methods Study of the Relationship between Food and Ethnic Identity in a Group of Mexican American Women," *Journal of the Academy of Nutrition and Dietetics* 118, no. 3 (March 2018): 431–39, https://doi.org/10.1016/j.jand.2017.10.008.

5. Jo Craven McGinty, "10,000 Steps a Day Is a Myth. The Number to Stay Healthy Is Far Lower," *Wall Street Journal,* June 12, 2020, https:// www.wsj.com/articles/10-000-steps-a-day-is-a-myth-the-number-to -stay-healthy-is-far-lower-11591968600.

6. I-Min Lee et al., "Association of Step Volume and Intensity with All-Cause Mortality in Older Women," *JAMA Internal*

Medicine 179, no. 8 (2019): 1,105–12, https://doi.org/10.1001/ja mainternmed.2019.0899.

Chapter Ten: Finding Body Acceptance

1. "Caroline Caldwell Quotes," GoodReads, n.d., https://www.go odreads.com/quotes/9371890-in-a-society-that-profits-from-your -self-doubt-liking.

2. Rene Germain, "Why We Need to Embrace Introverted Black Women in the Workplace," *Cosmopolitan*, October 21, 2021, https://www .cosmopolitan.com/uk/worklife/careers/a37999565/introverted-black -women-workplace/.

3. Lindsay Kramer, "What Is a Straw Man Argument? Definition and Examples," Grammarly, June 2, 2022, https://www.grammarly.com /blog/straw-man-fallacy/.

4. Andrea Gordon, "Did You Ever Realize," Mind Journal, n.d., https:// themindsjournal.com/quotes/did-you-ever-realize-how-much-your -body-loves-you/.

5. Dr. Kristin Neff, "Definition of Self-Compassion," Self-Compassion .org, n.d., https://self-compassion.org/the-three-elements-of-self-com passion-2/.

6. Gary Goldfield, PhD, "Reducing Social Media Use Significantly Improves Body Image in Teens, Young Adults," American Psychological Association, February 23, 2023, https://www.apa.org/news/press/re leases/2023/02/social-media-body-image.

7. Clarissa Silva, "Social Media's Impact on Self-Esteem," *HuffPost*, February 22, 2017, https://www.huffpost.com/entry/social-medias-im pact-on-self-esteem_b_58ade038e4b0d818c4f0a4e4.

8. Alli Patton, "Megan Thee Stallion Launches Site Compiling Mental Health Resources for Fans," American Songwriter, September 27, 2022, https://americansongwriter.com/megan-thee-stallion-launches -site-compiling-mental-health-resources-for-fans/.

INDEX

ABOUT THE AUTHOR

Shana Spence is a Registered Dietitian Nutritionist based in New York. She is an "all foods fit" dietitian. Life is already complicated; why restrict yourself unnecessarily? She creates a platform for open discussion on nutrition and wellness topics that are anti-diet, Health at Every Size, and non–weight centric related, considering all the information circulating these days. Was she always interested in nutrition? No. In the not-so-long-ago past, she worked in the fashion industry and hated it. (The joke is, she got a BS in Fashion Merchandising . . . get it?) She finally decided to make a change, went back to school, and became involved in food policy and public health, where she currently works. In addition to this, she owns her business, The Nutrition Tea, which provides consulting and counseling work.

Speaking engagements include Peloton, NEDA, Eating Recovery Center, The Rose Retreats, Food Fluence 2022, and Eat Well Global. She can be seen in media such as NPR, *Shape* magazine, *GQ, SELF* magazine, *Women's Health* magazine, *Outside* magazine, *Good Morning America*, and Healthline.

Podcasts include *Conversations with Kenzie, Well and Good, Train Happy Podcast, The Light Show, Real Pod, Let Us Eat Cake, What the Actual Fork*, and *RD Real Talk*.